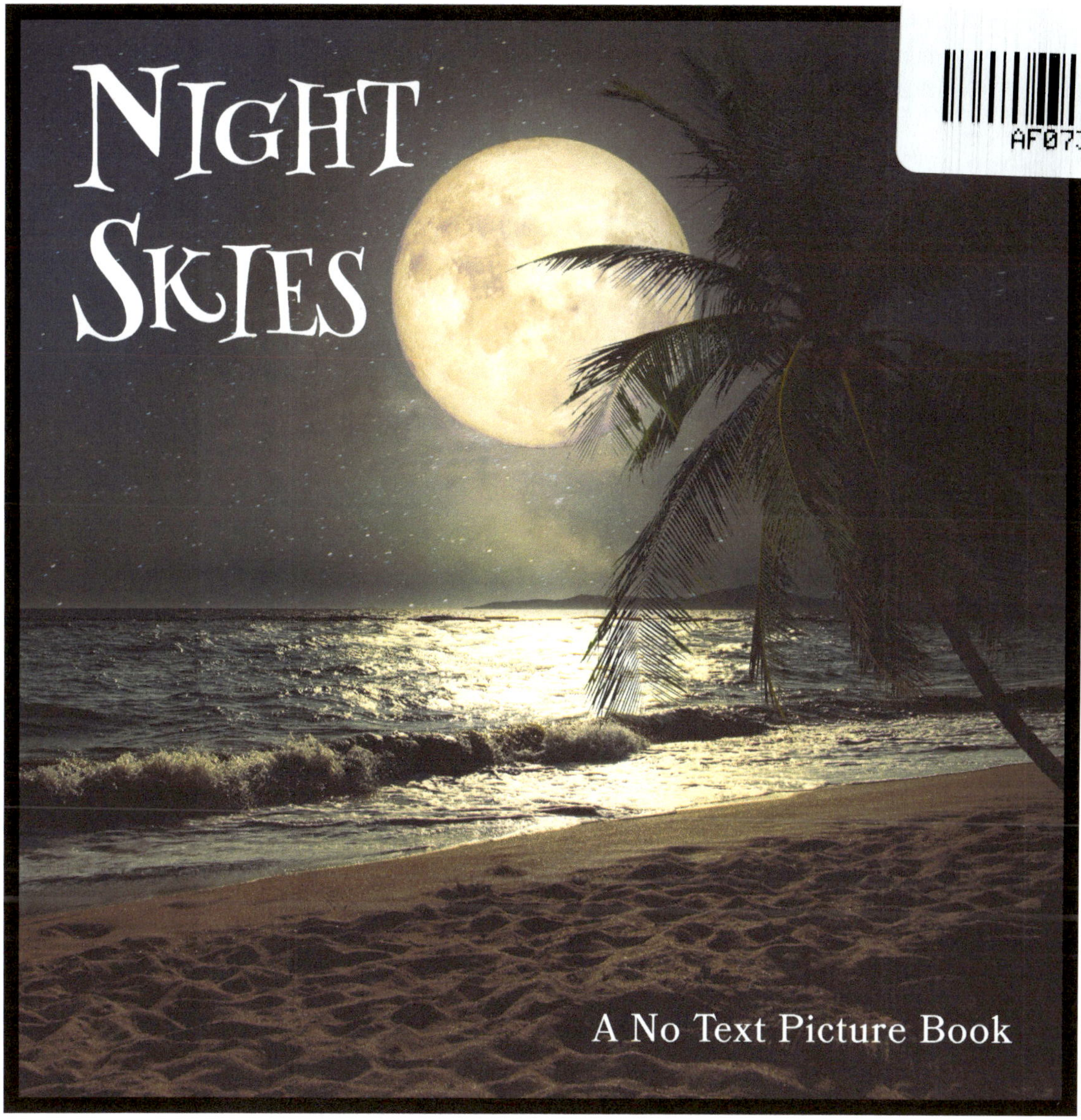
NIGHT
SKIES
A No Text Picture Book

AF073845

© 2021 Lasting Happiness | All rights reserved.
No part of this book may be reproduced or copied in any manner without prior written permission from the publisher.

ISBN: 9798744938901

To:

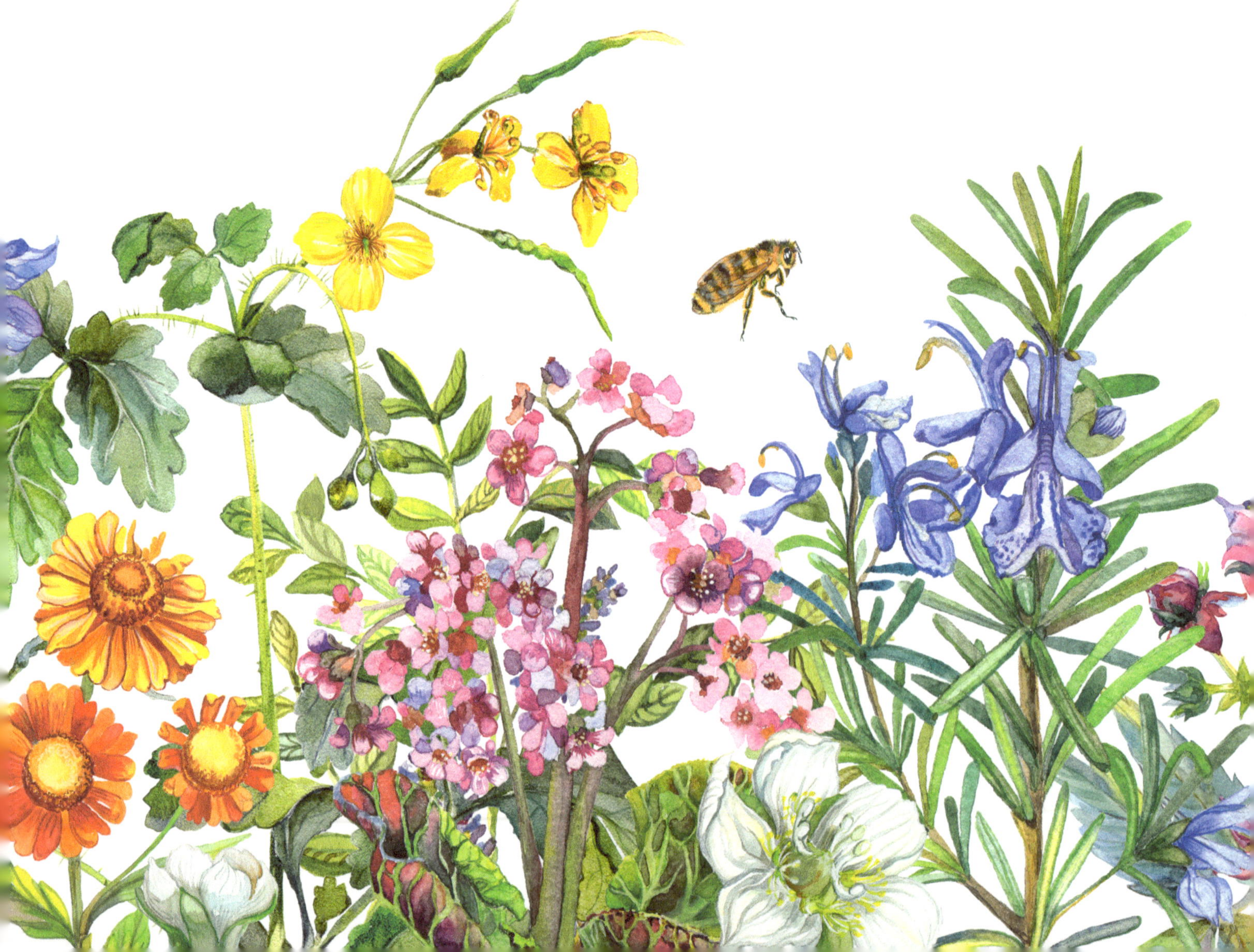

FROM:

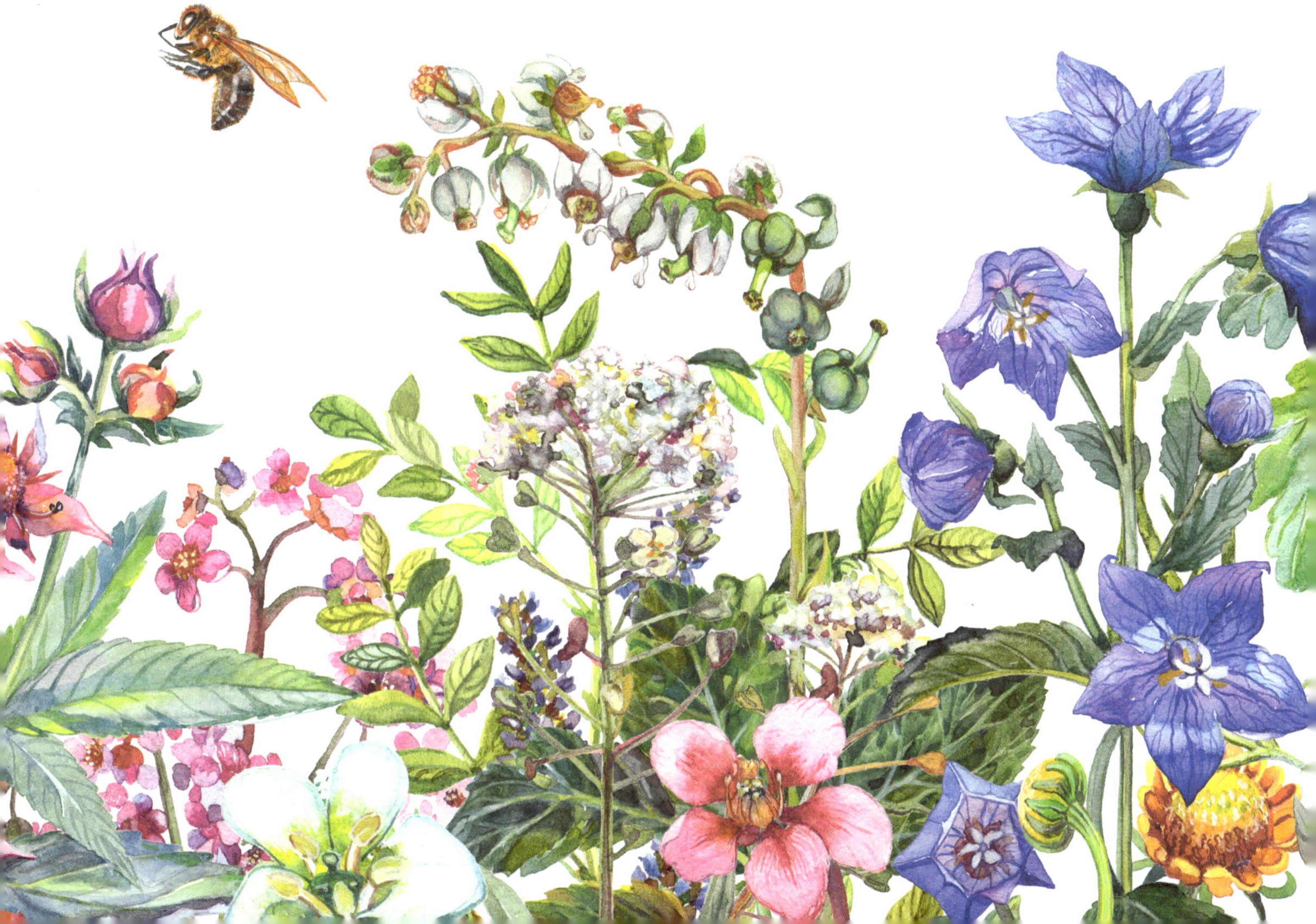

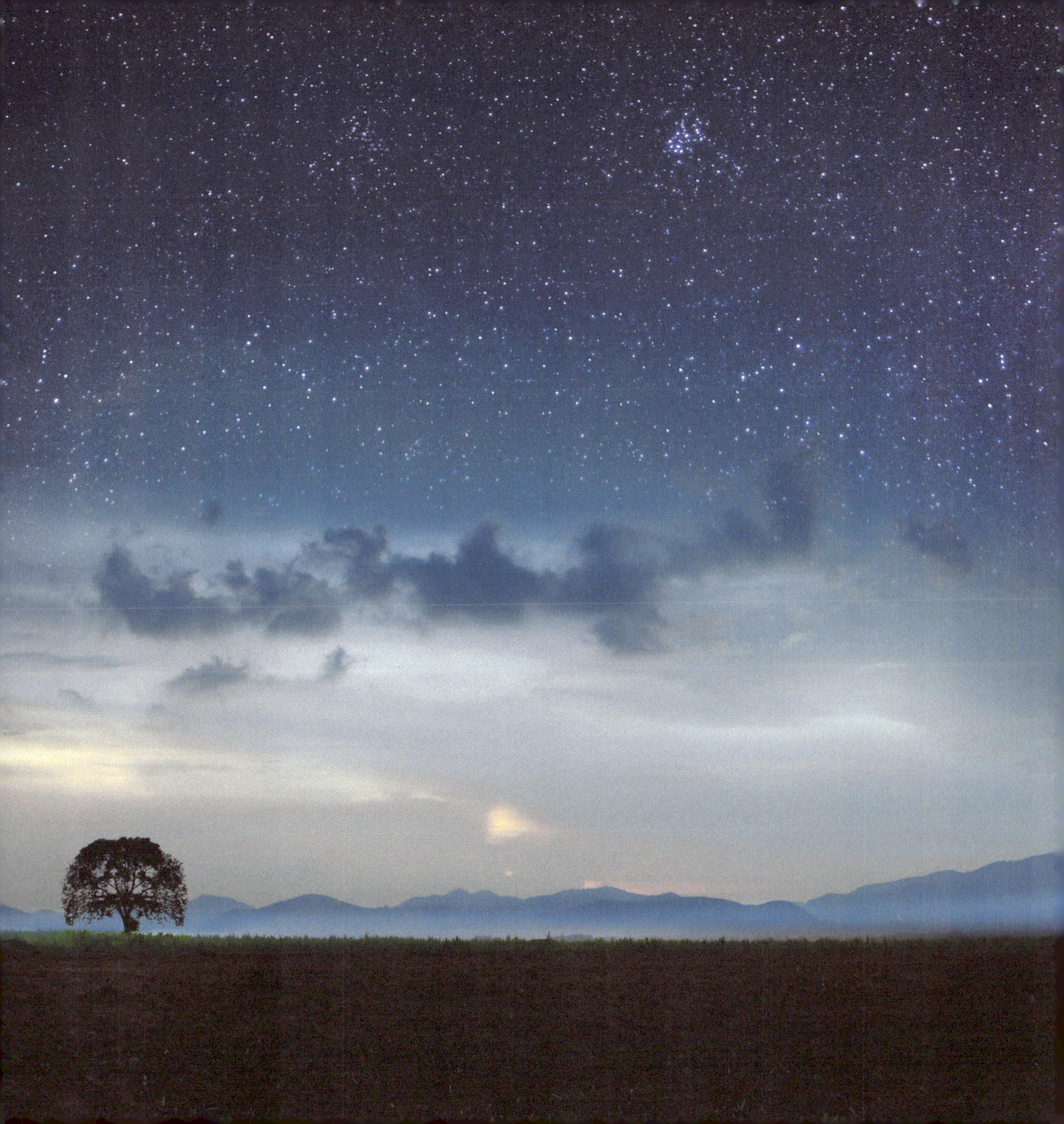

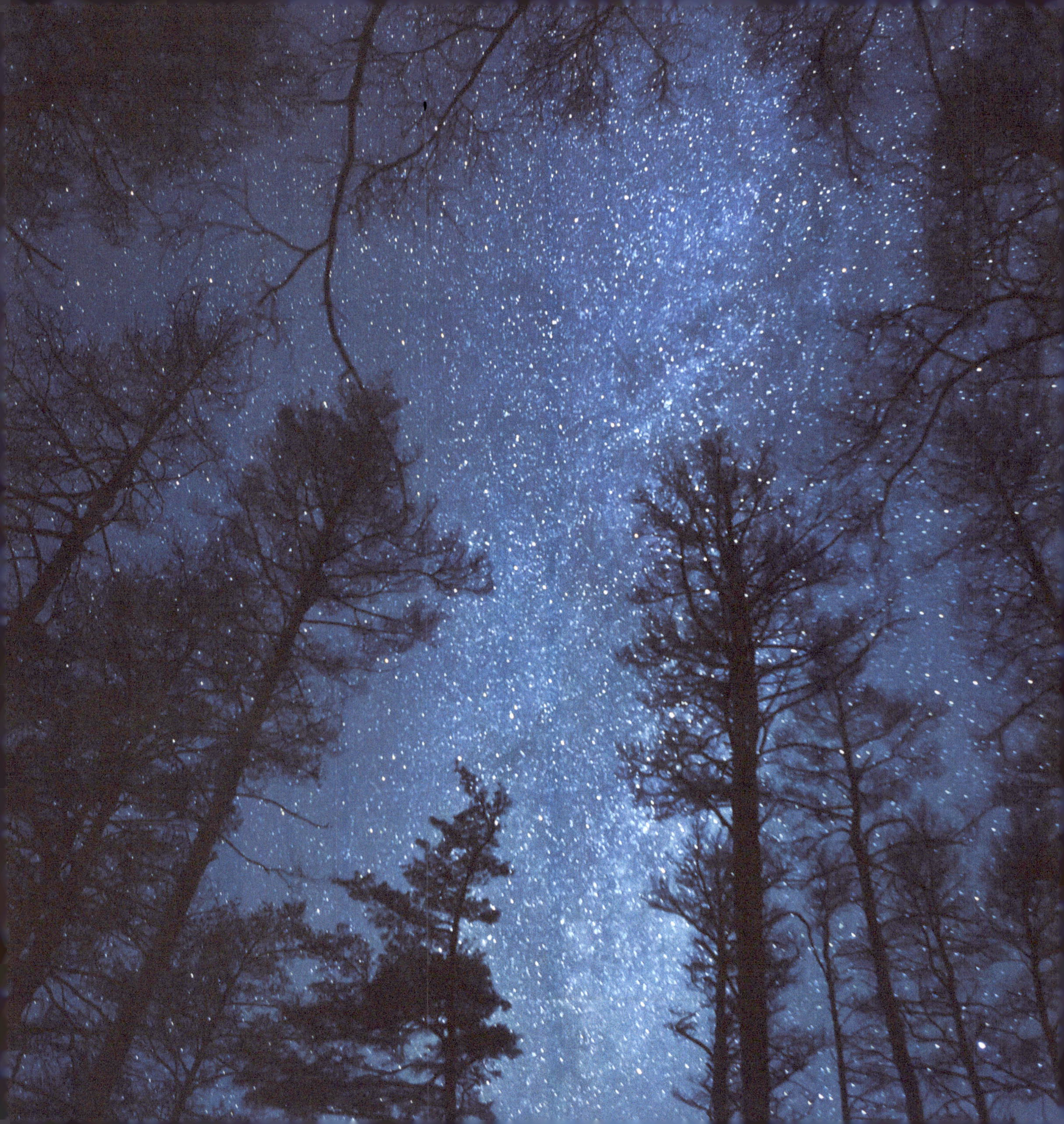

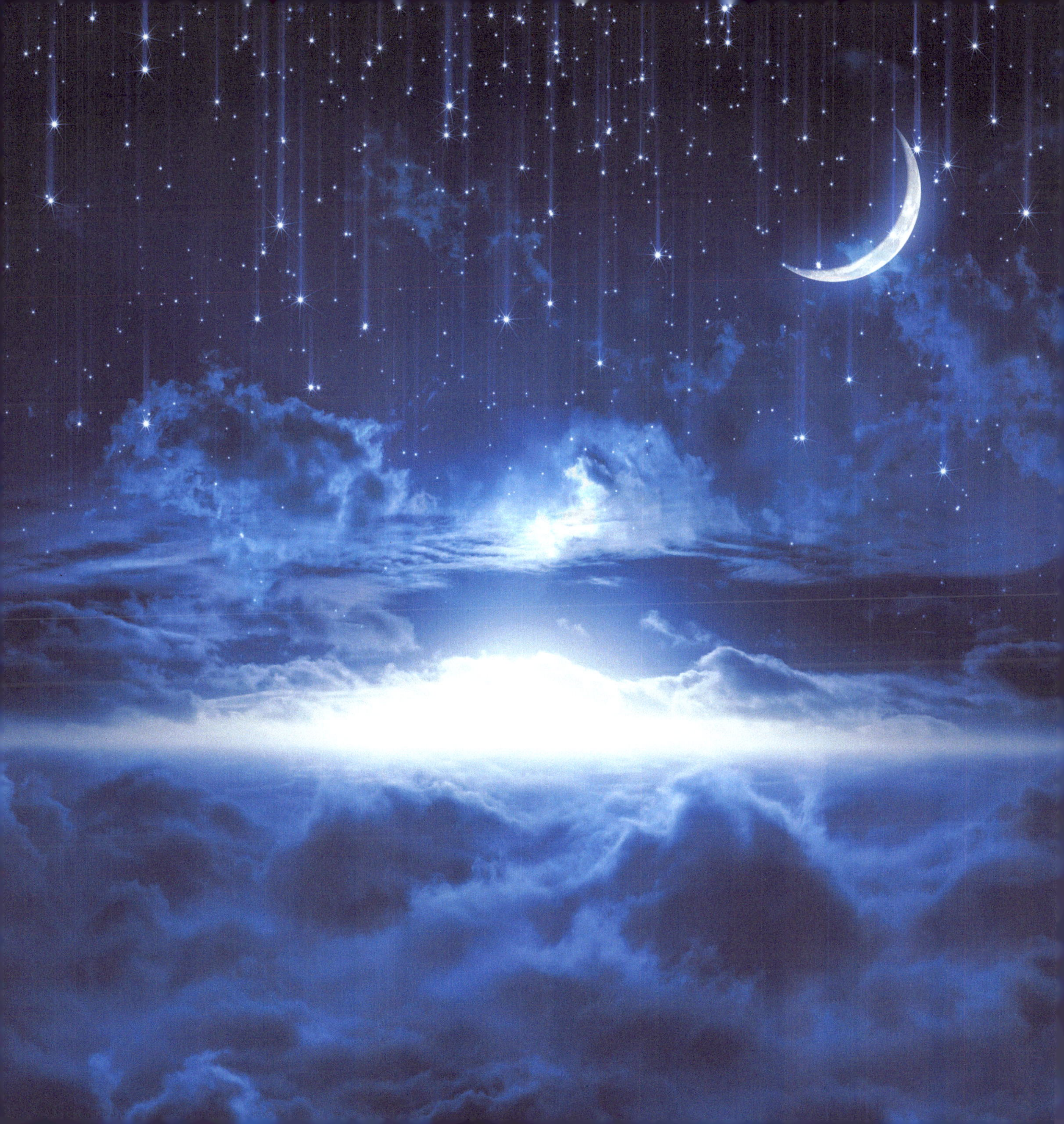

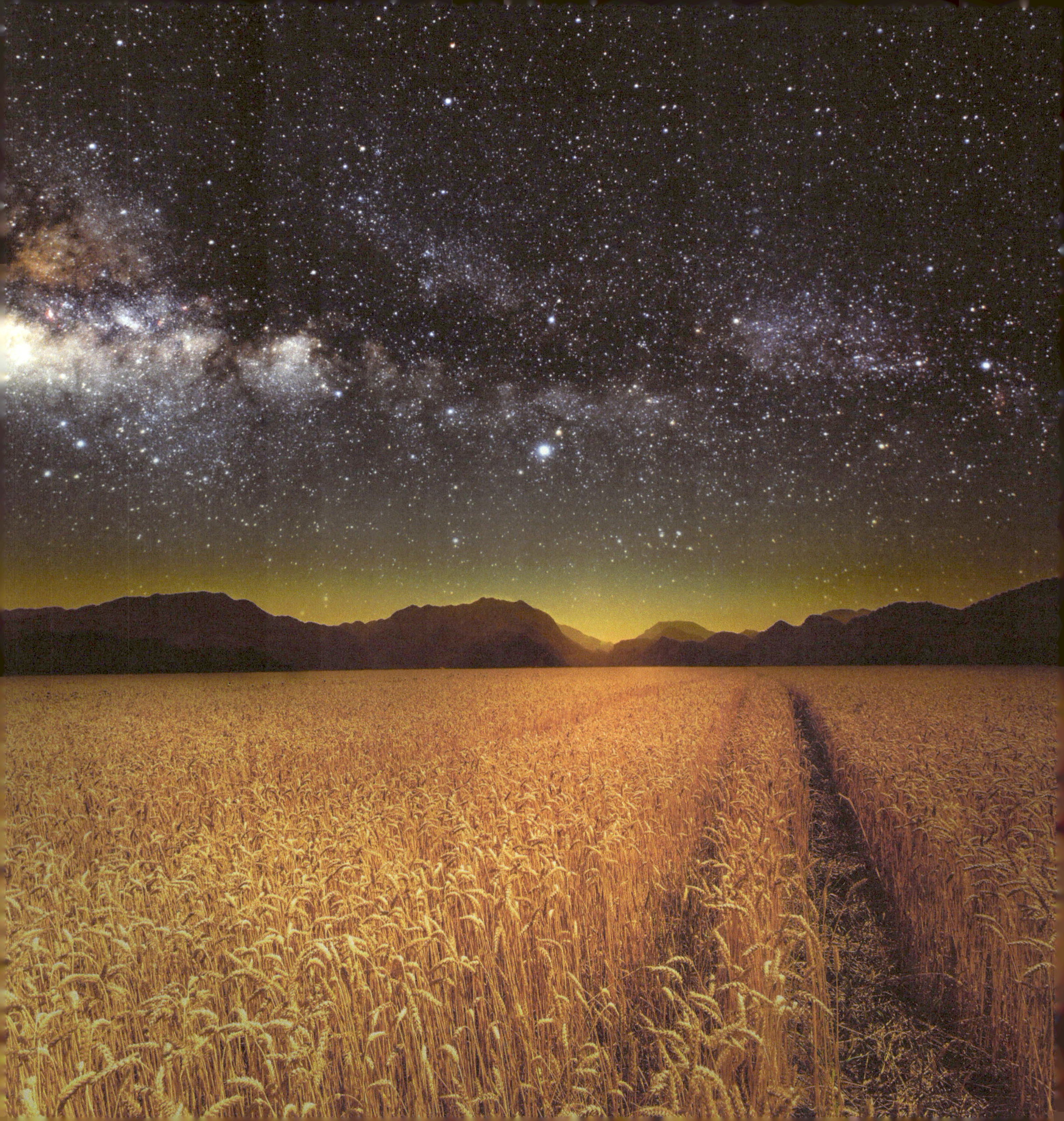

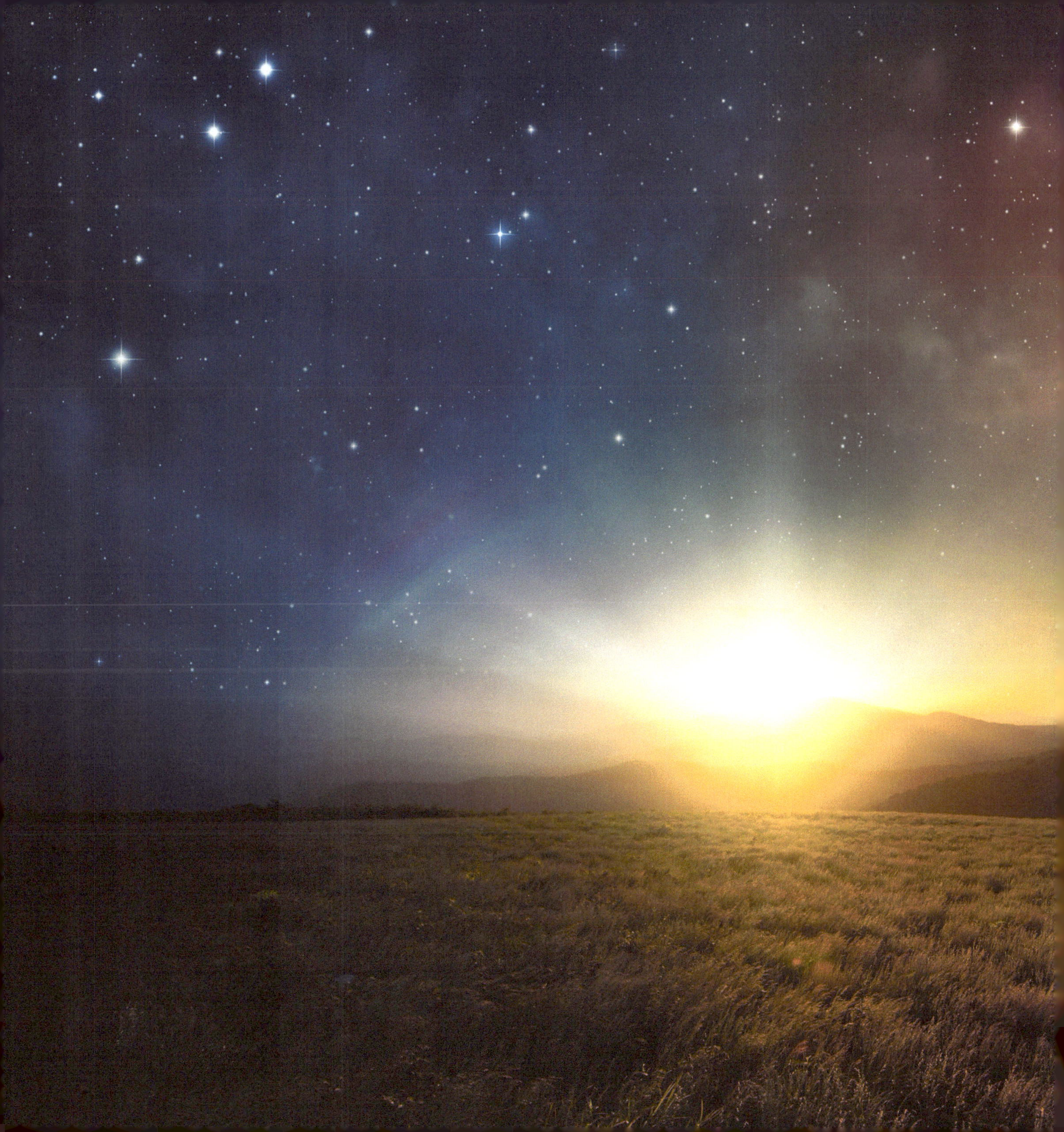

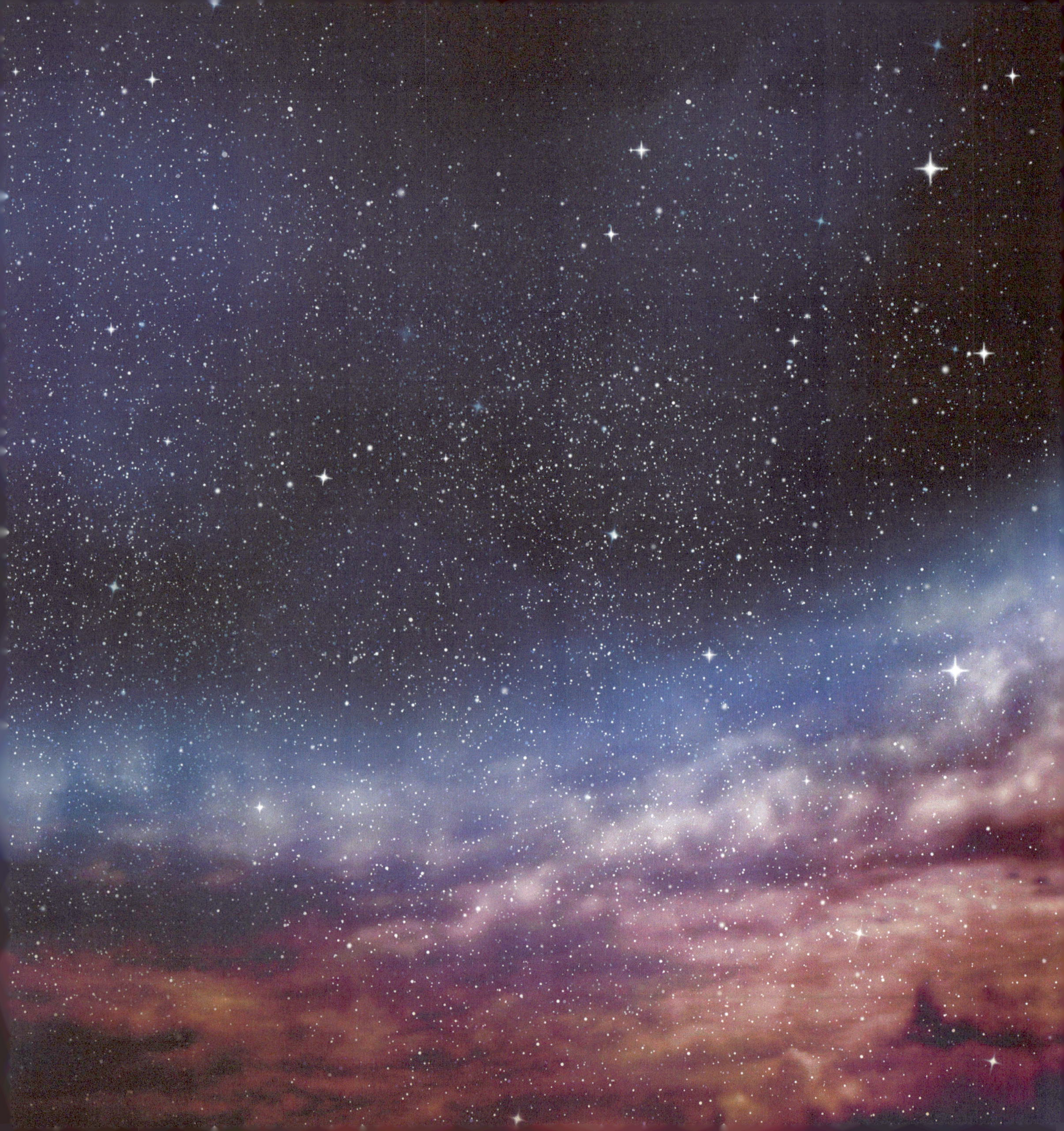

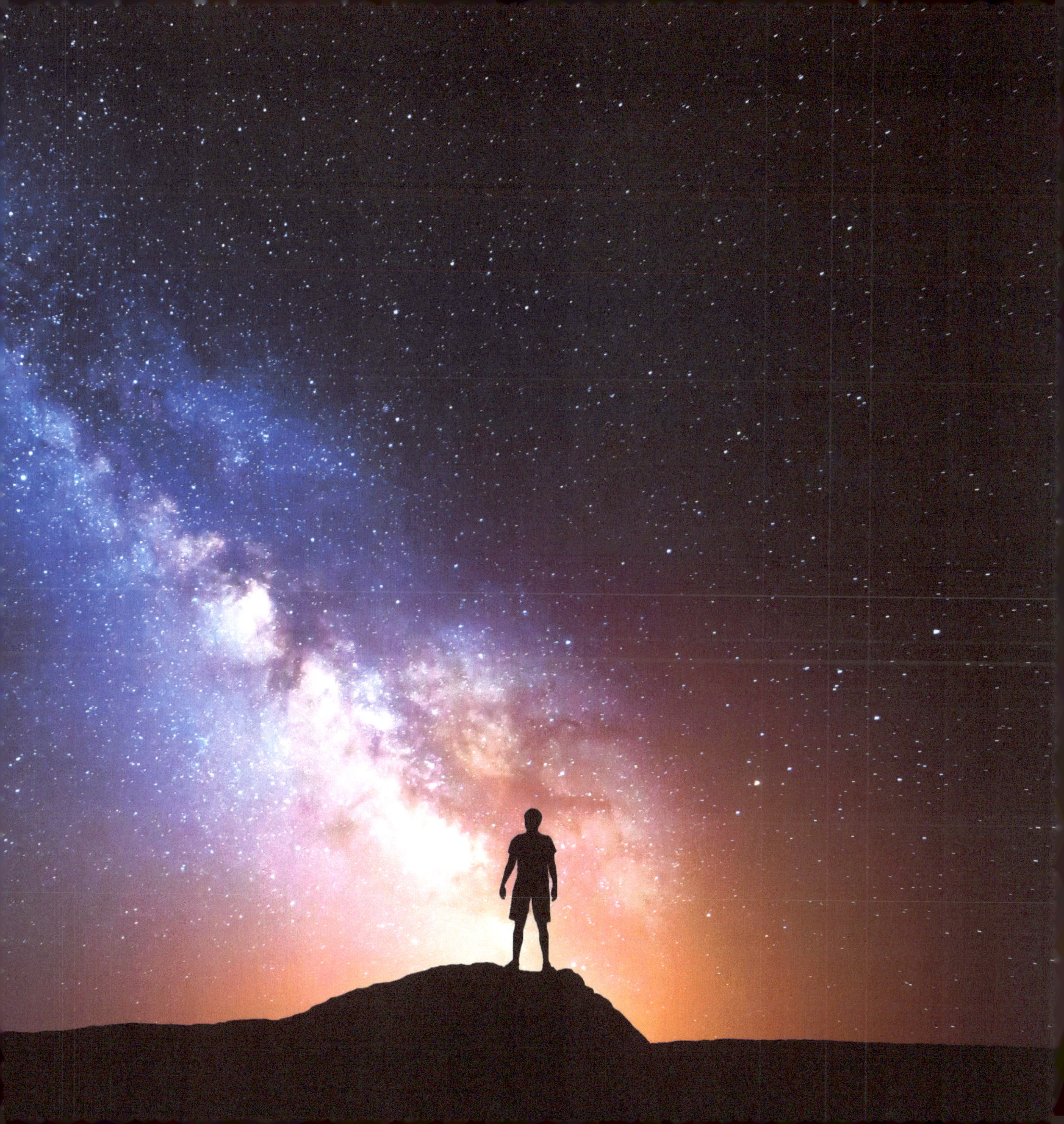

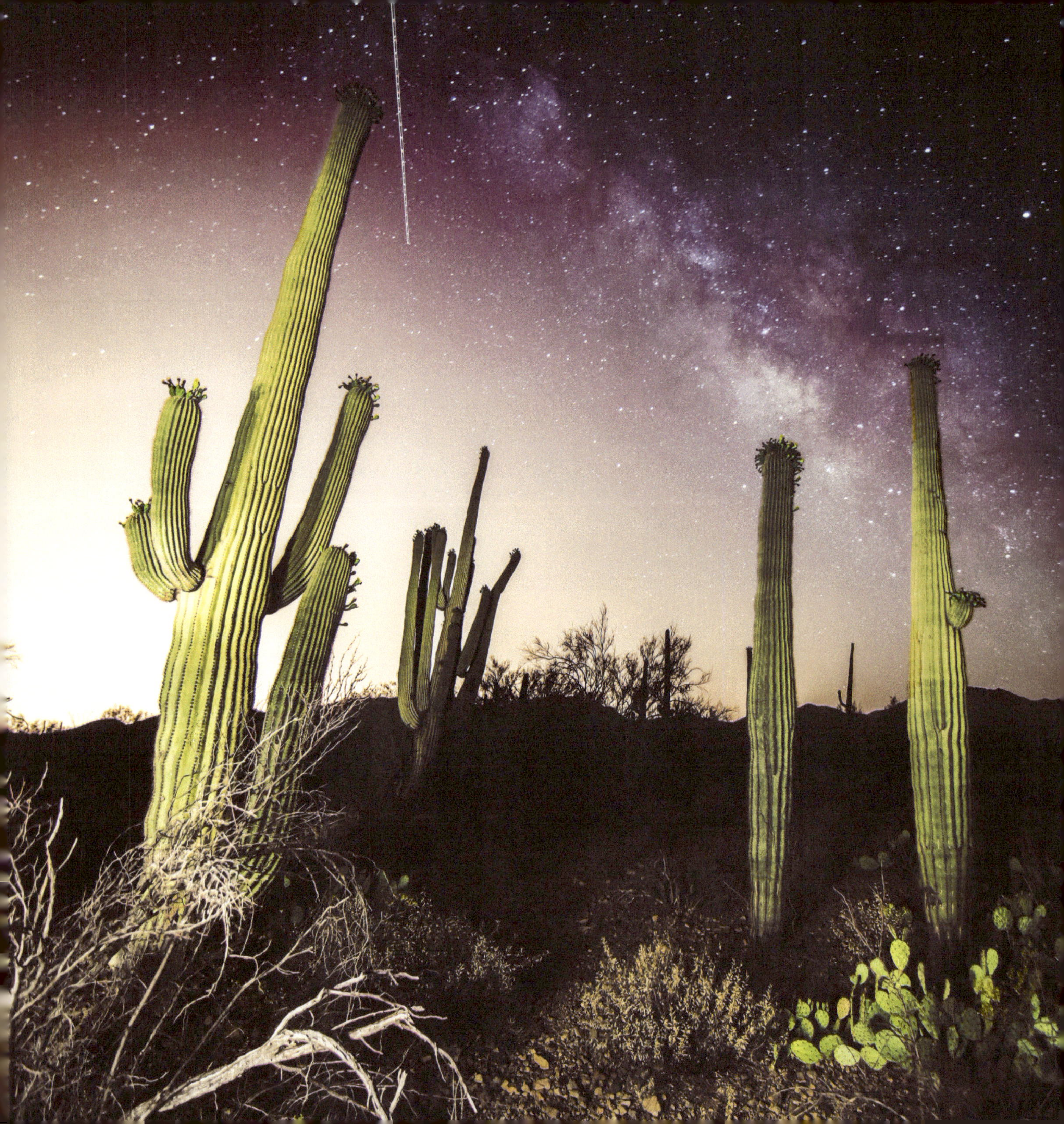

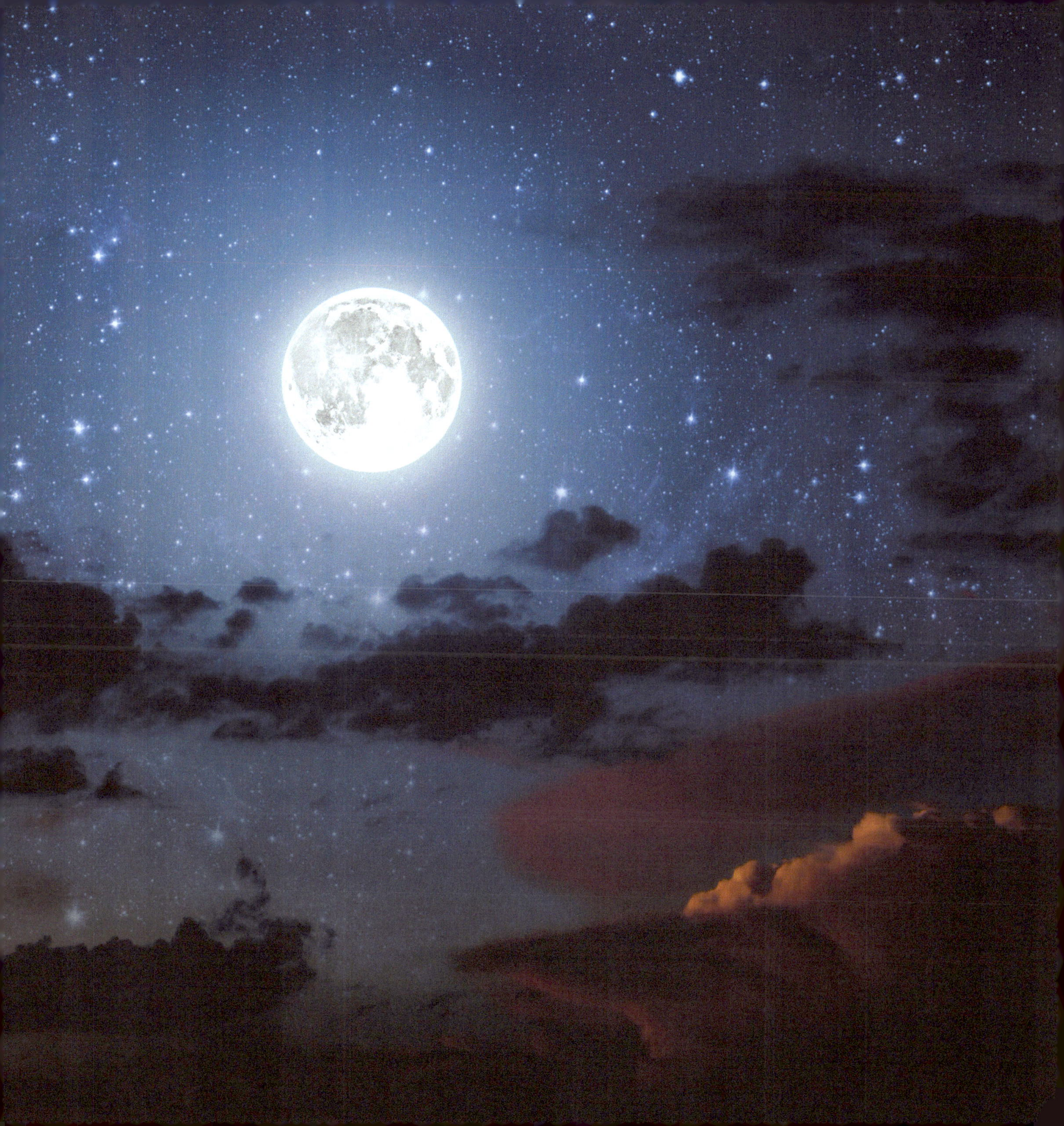

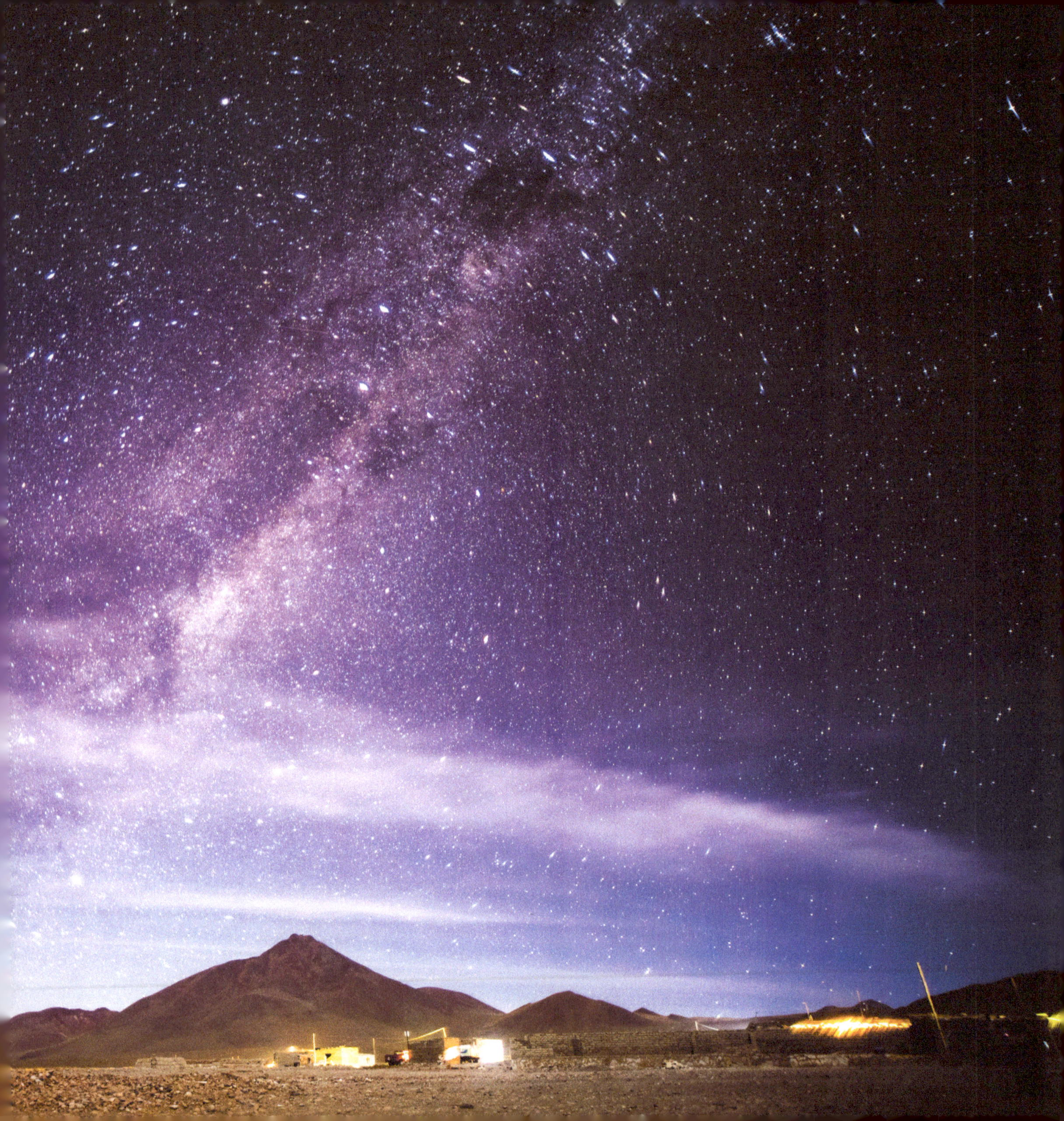

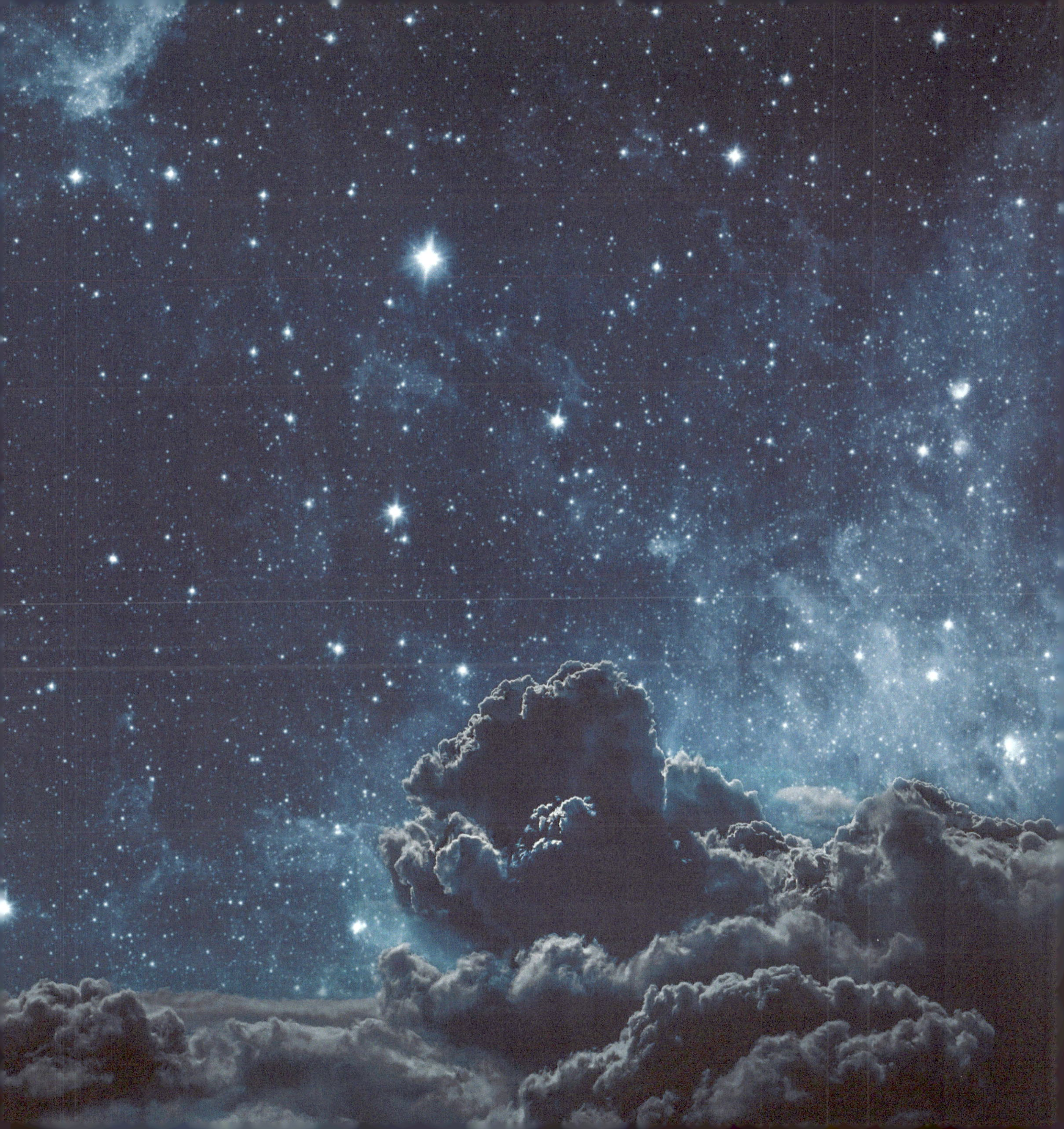

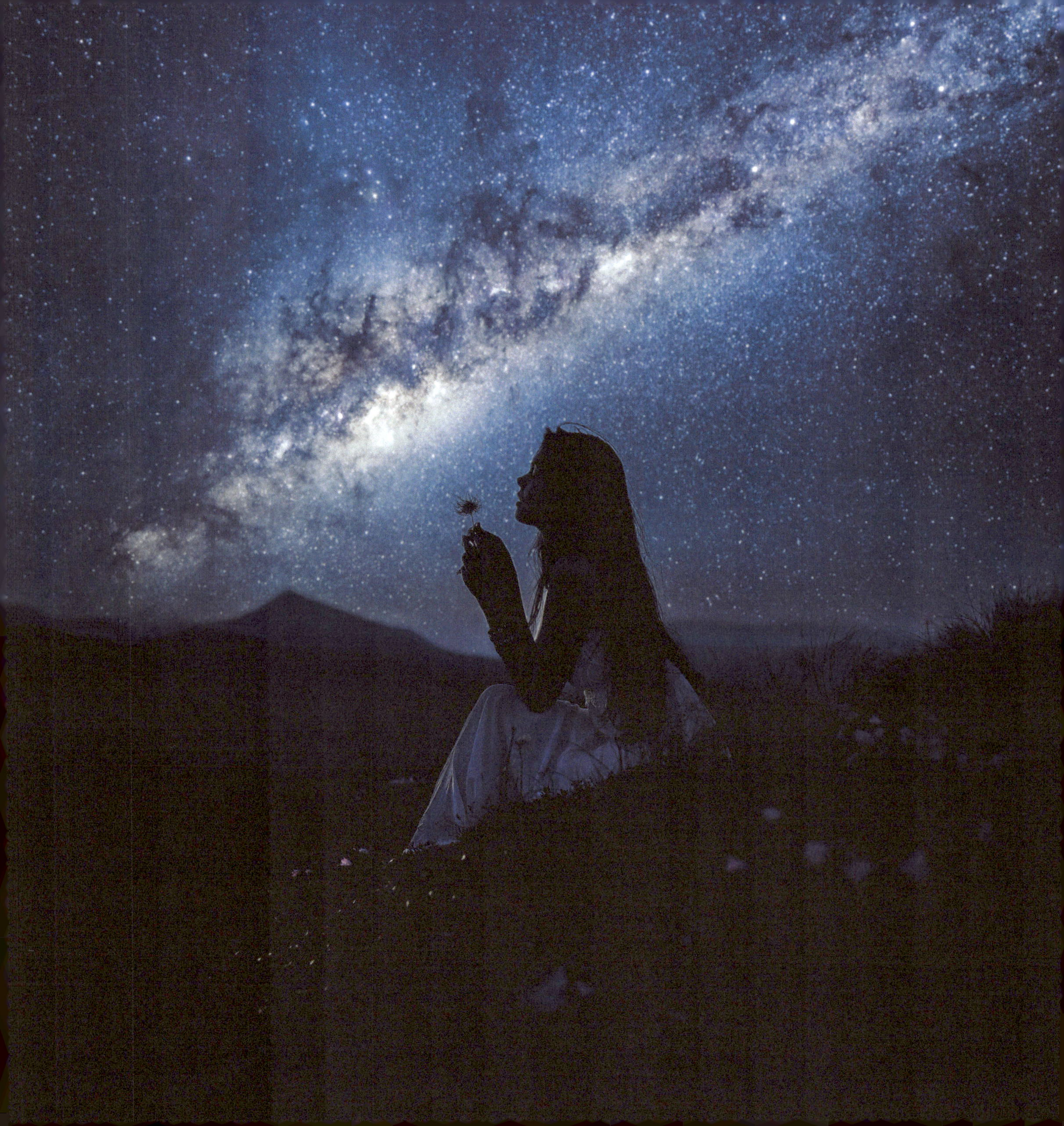

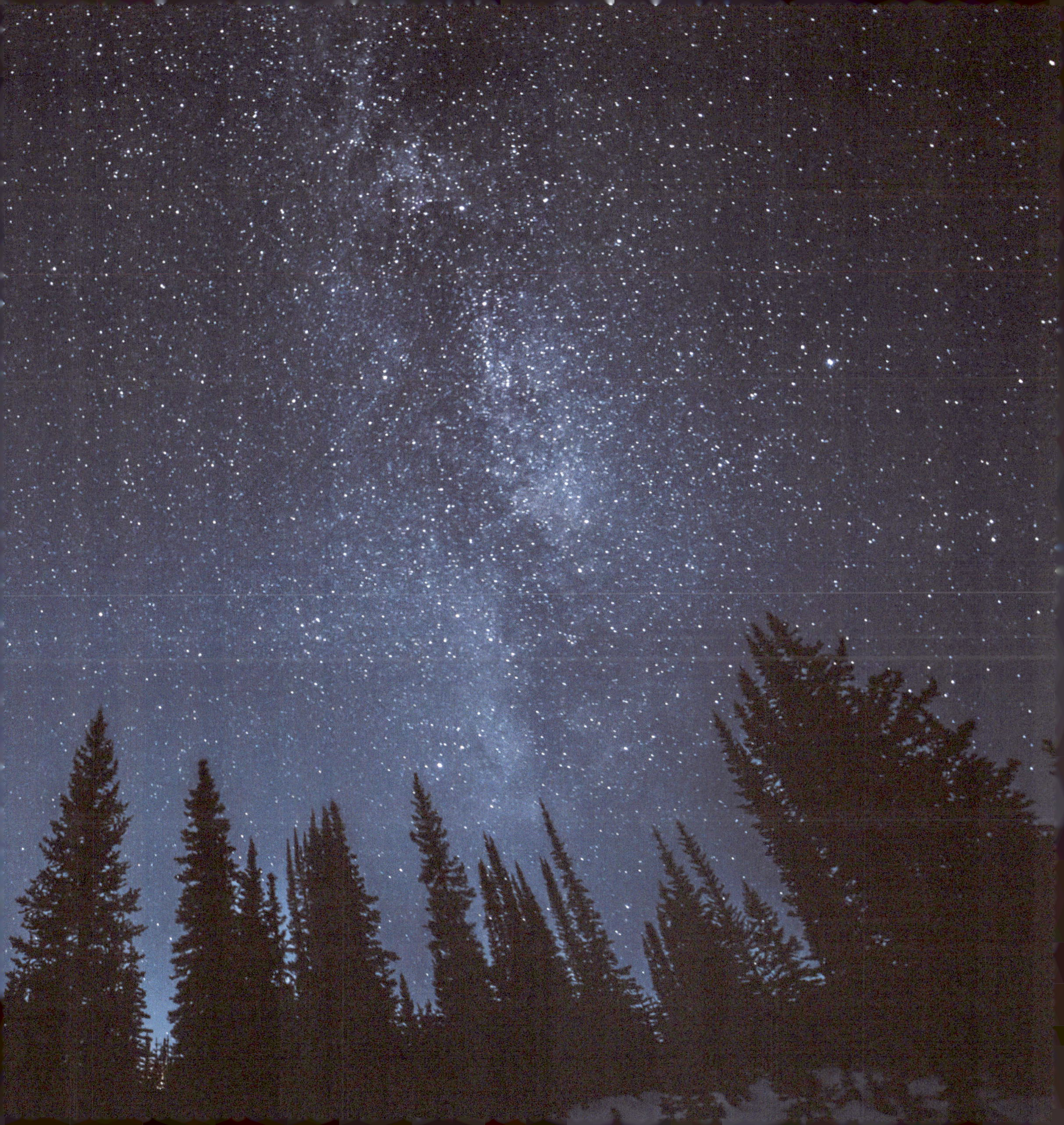

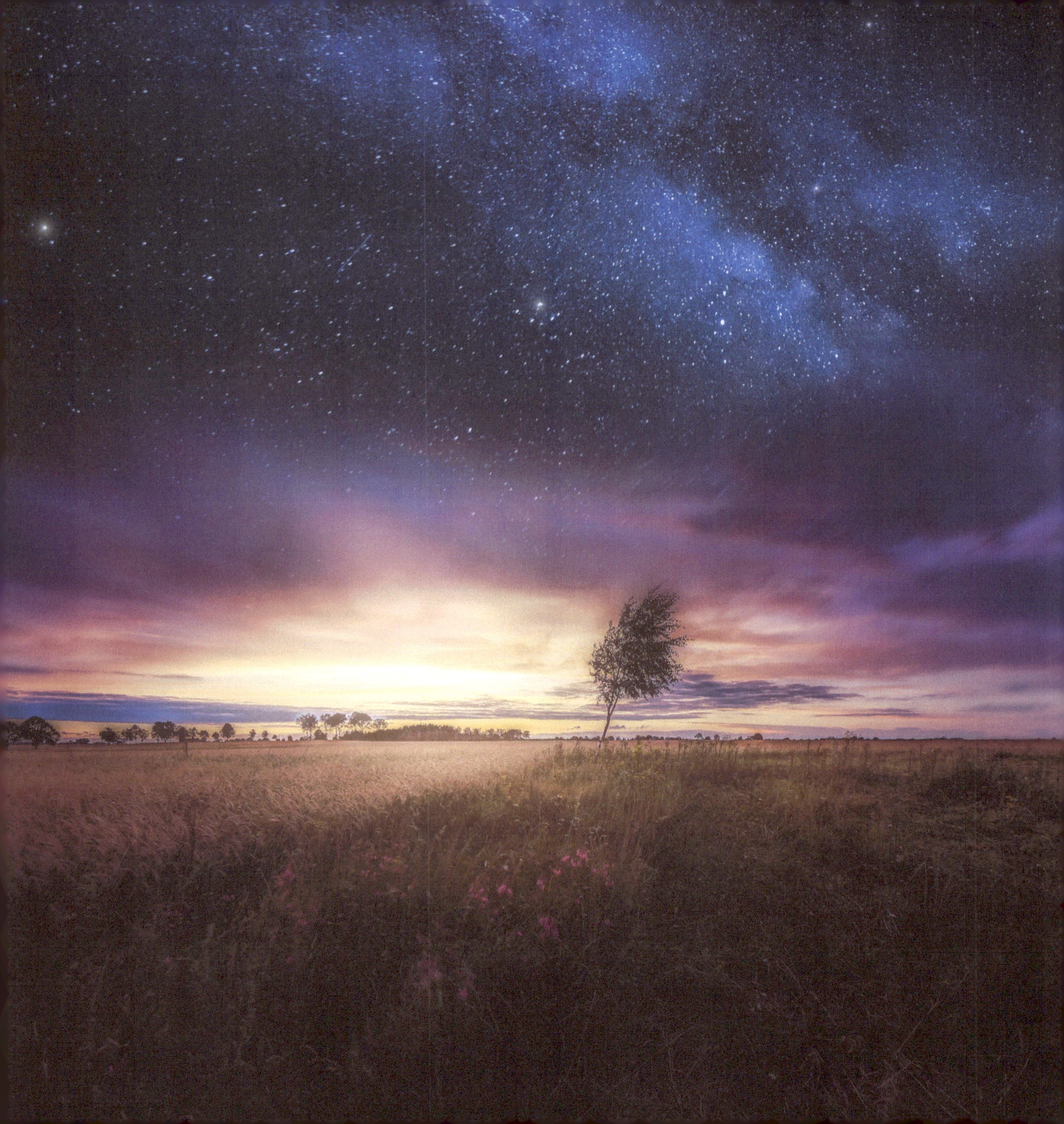

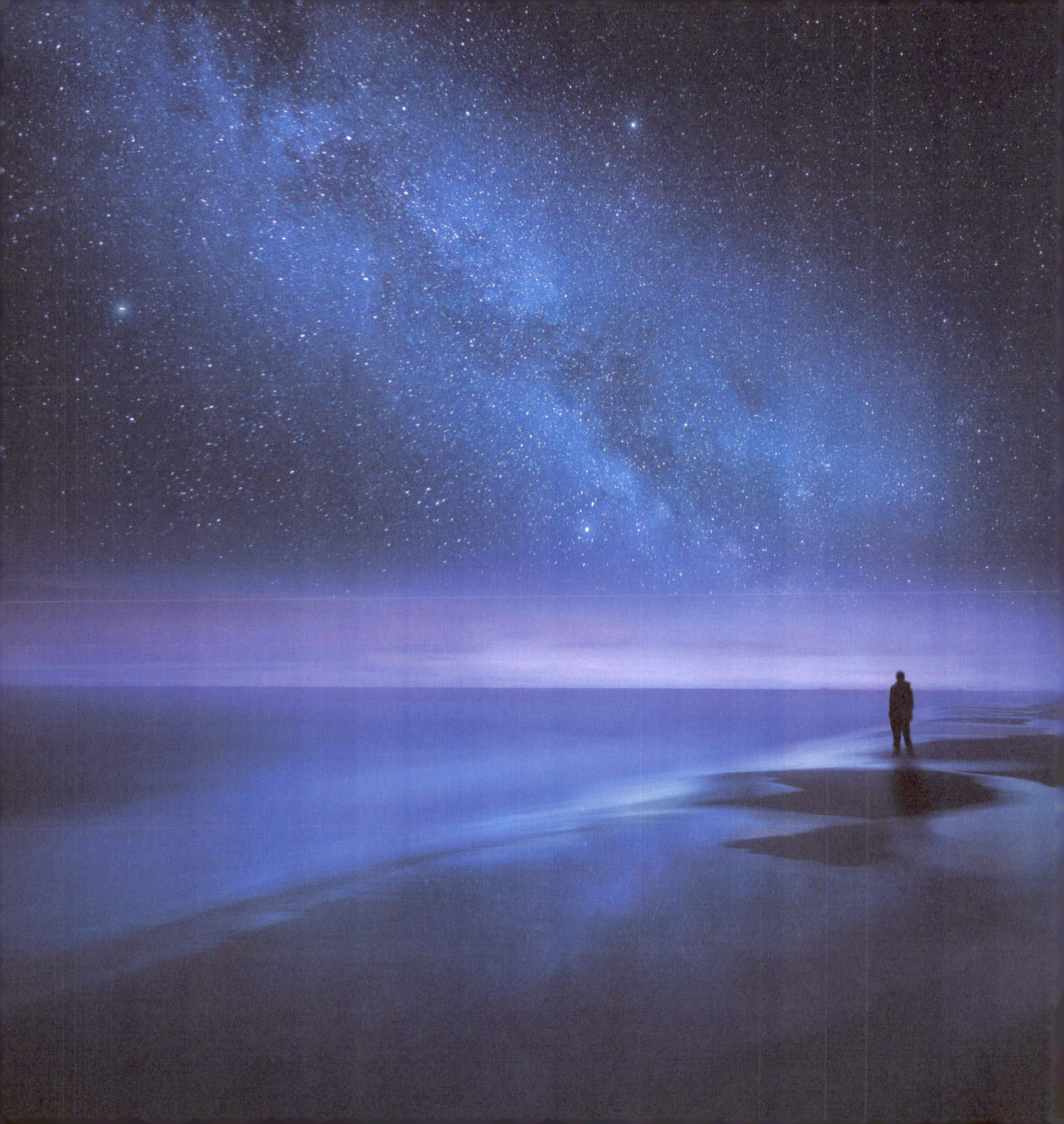

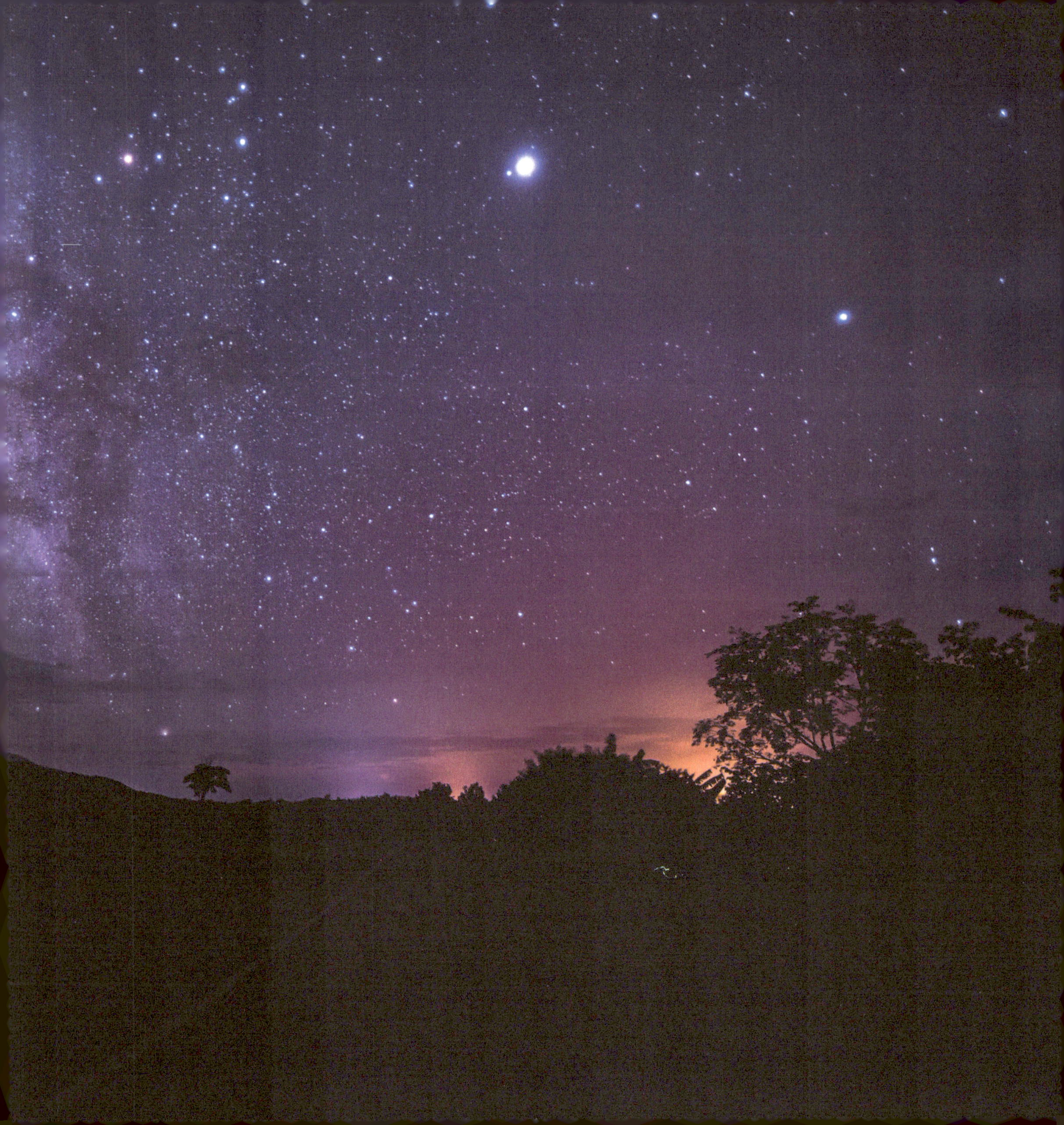

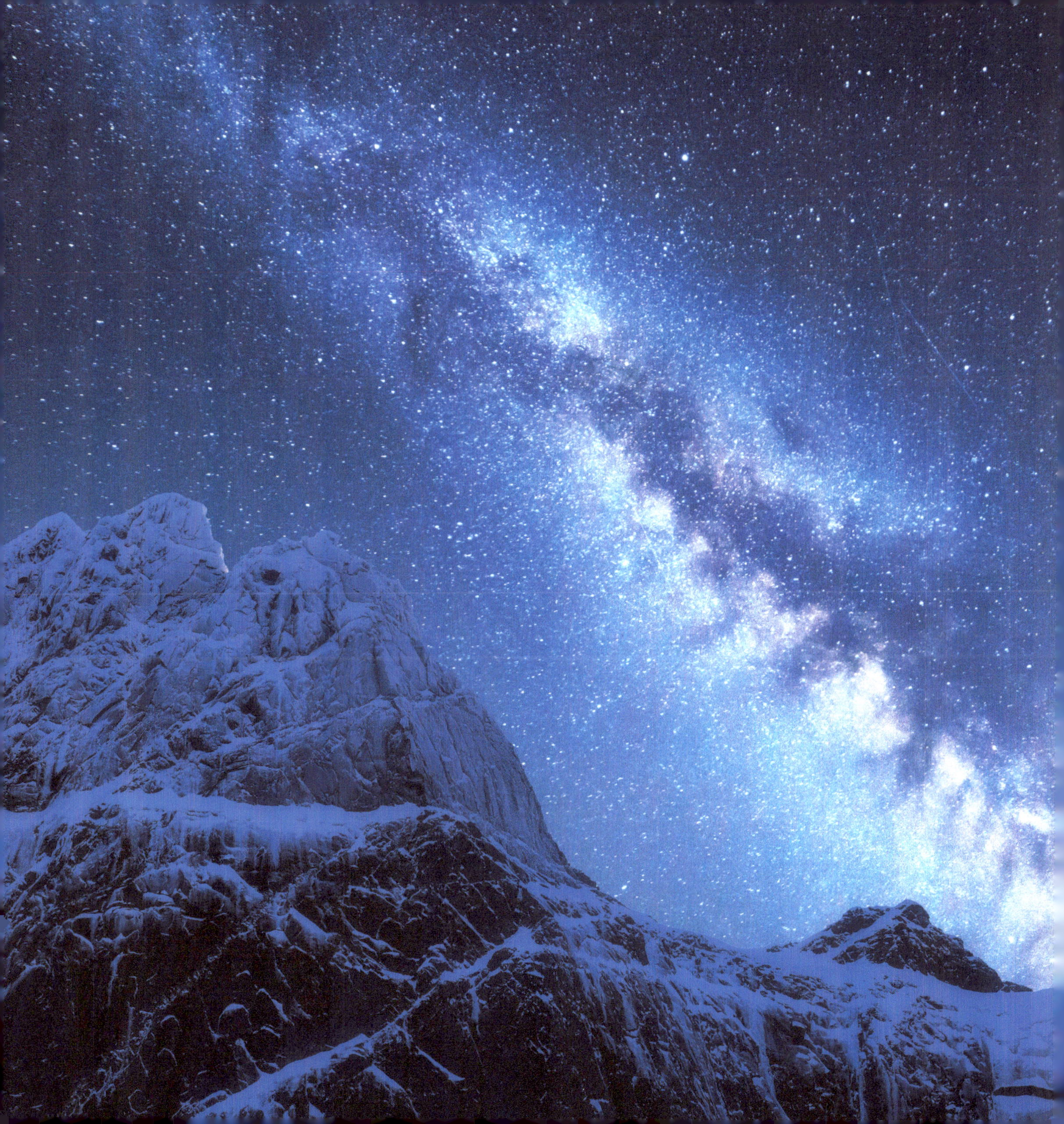

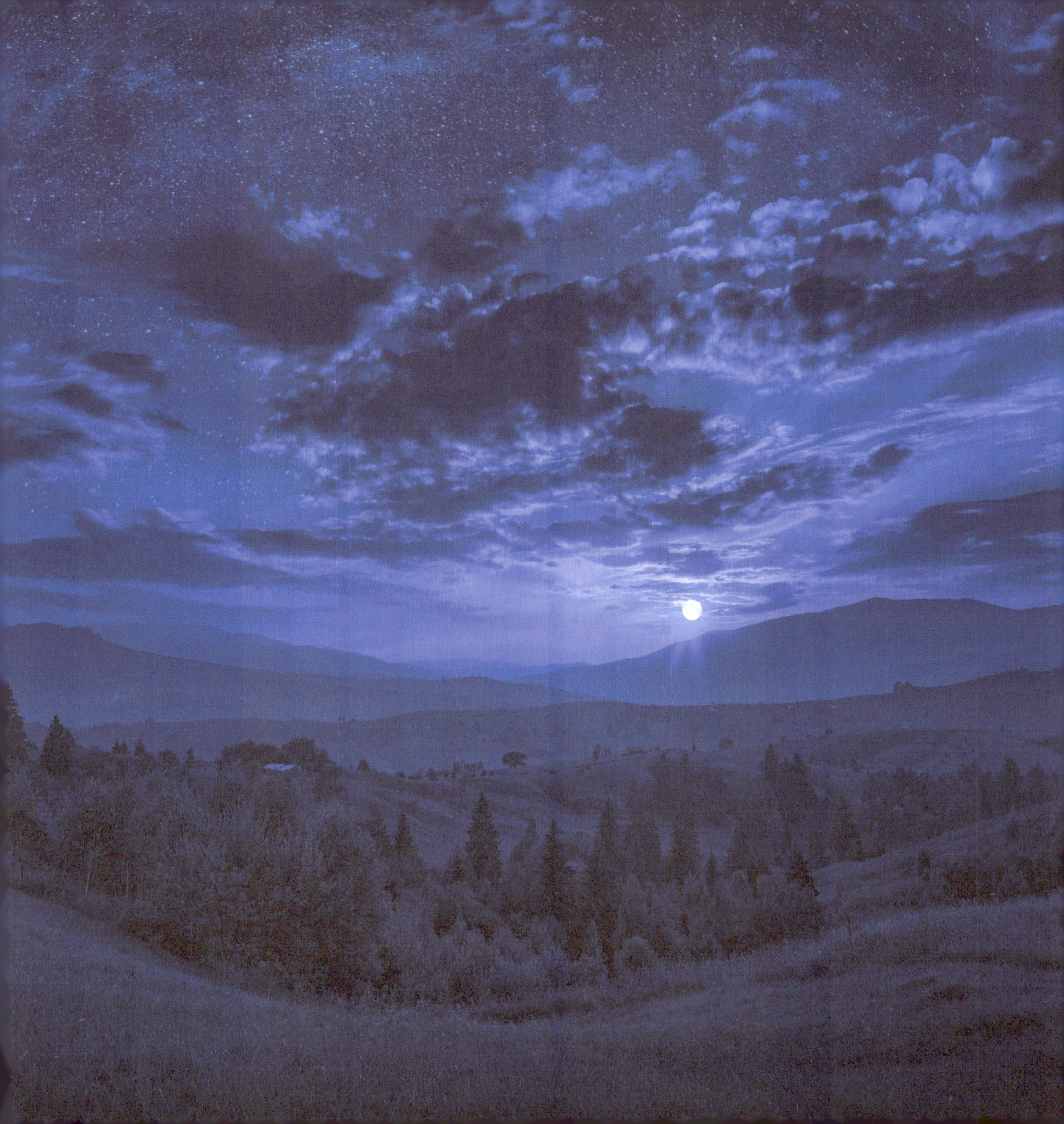

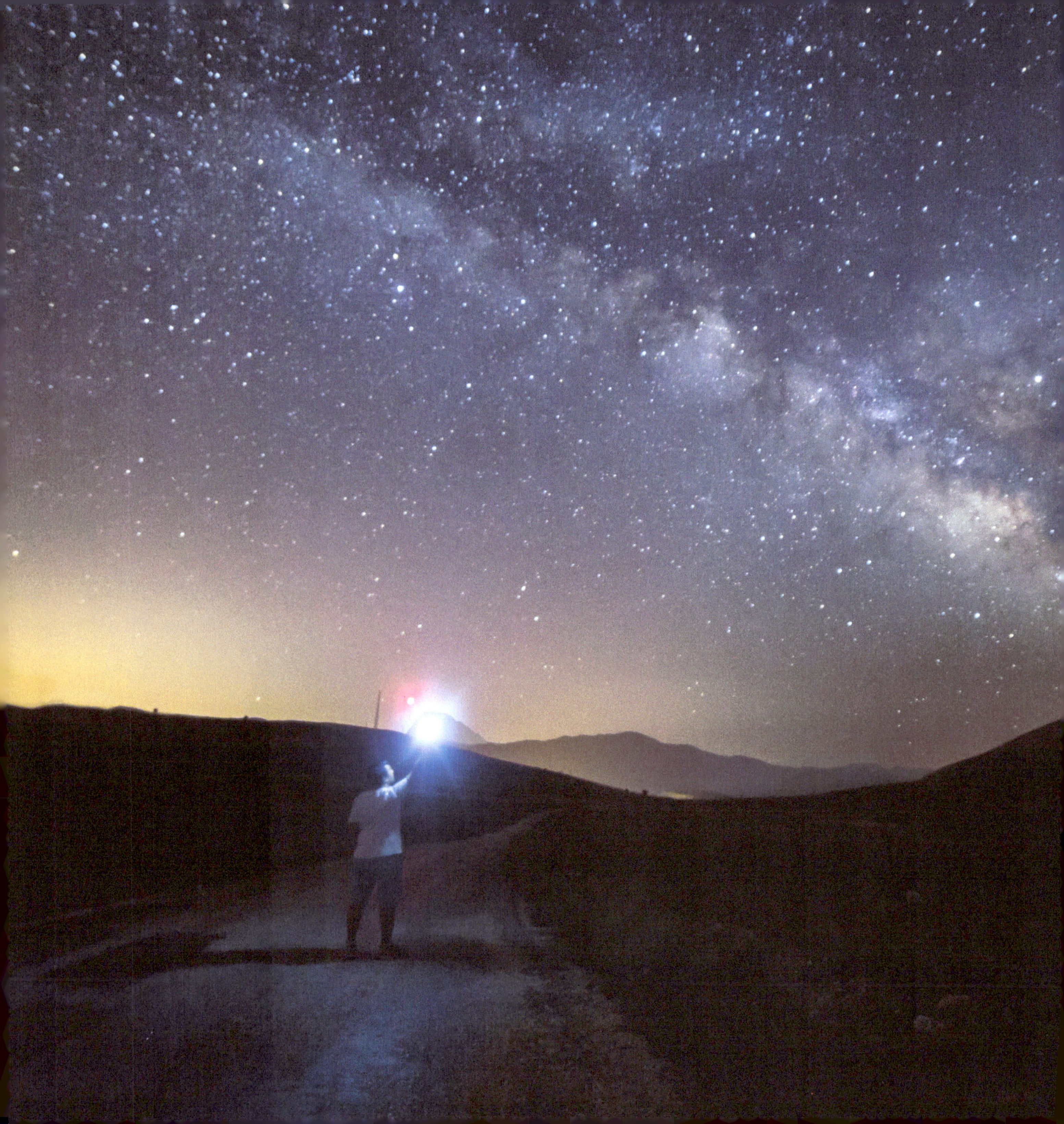

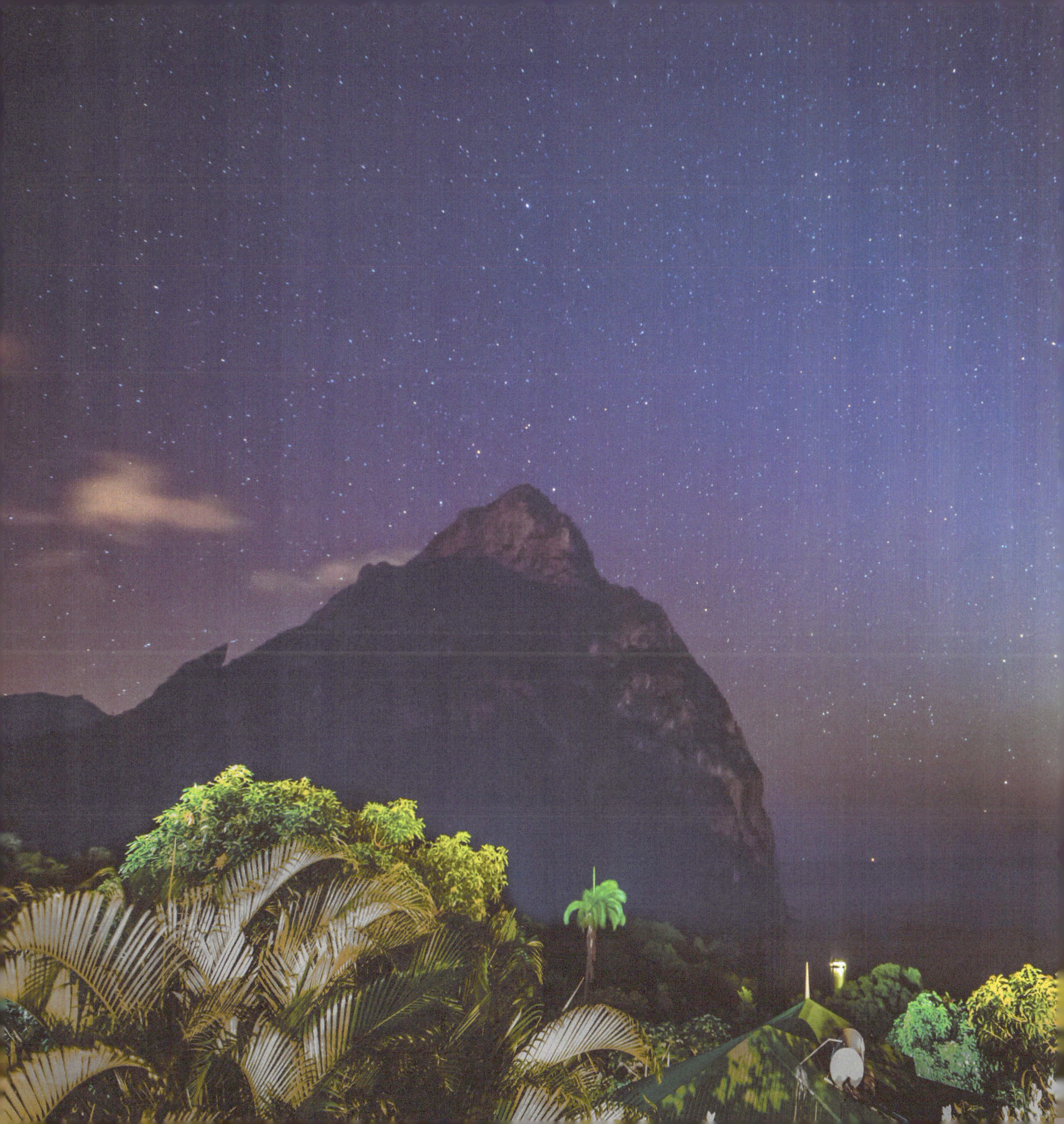

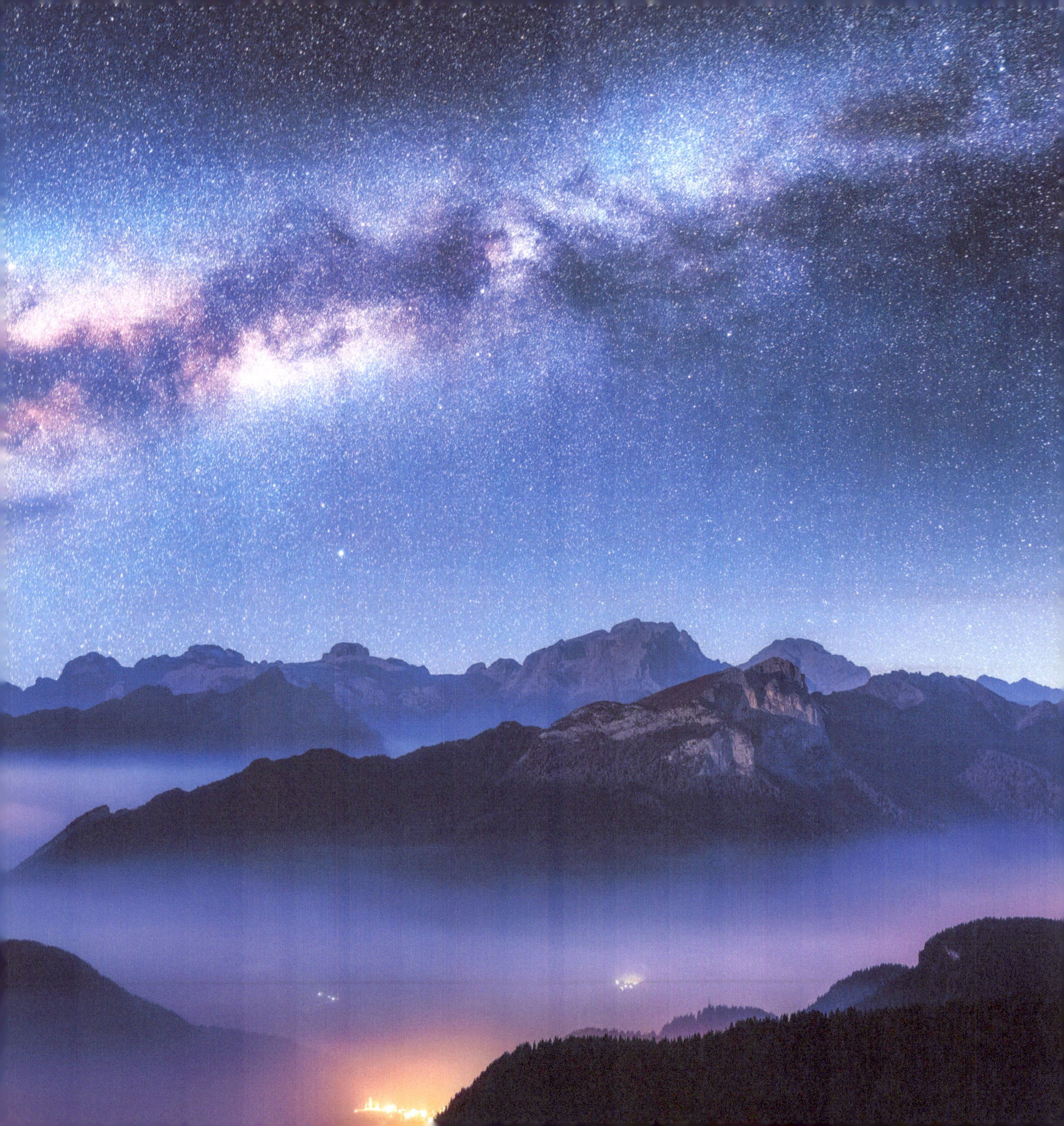

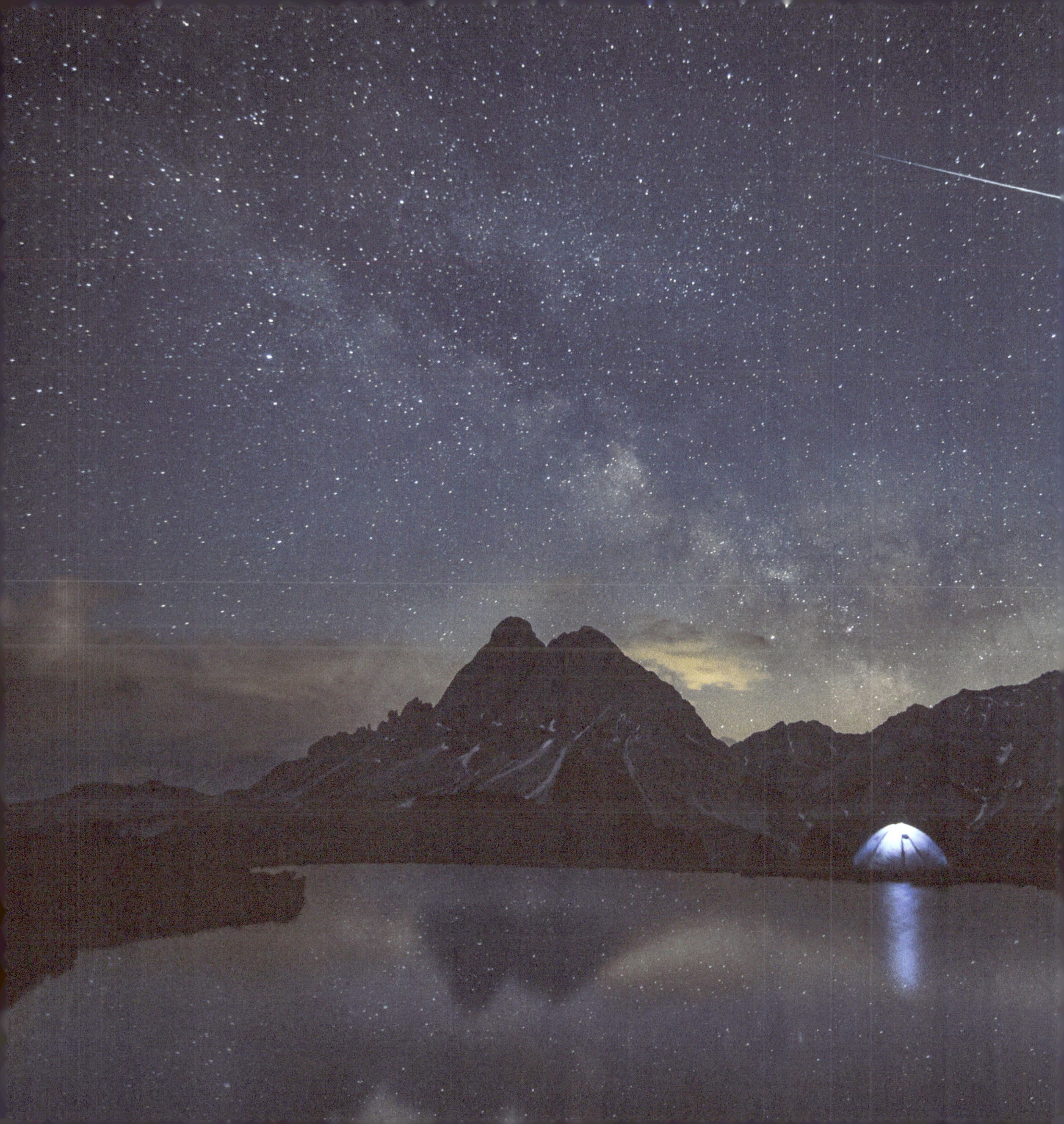

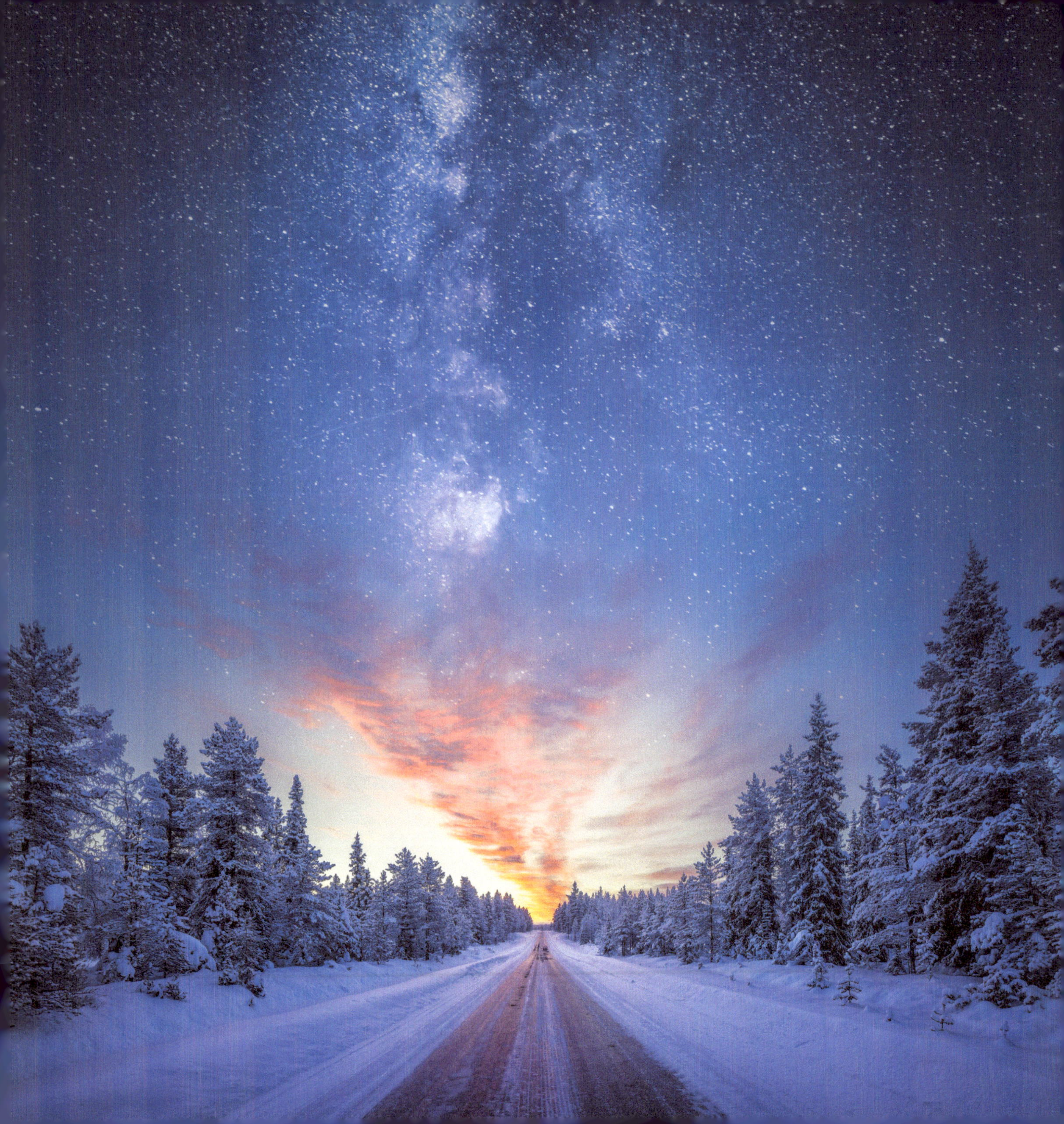

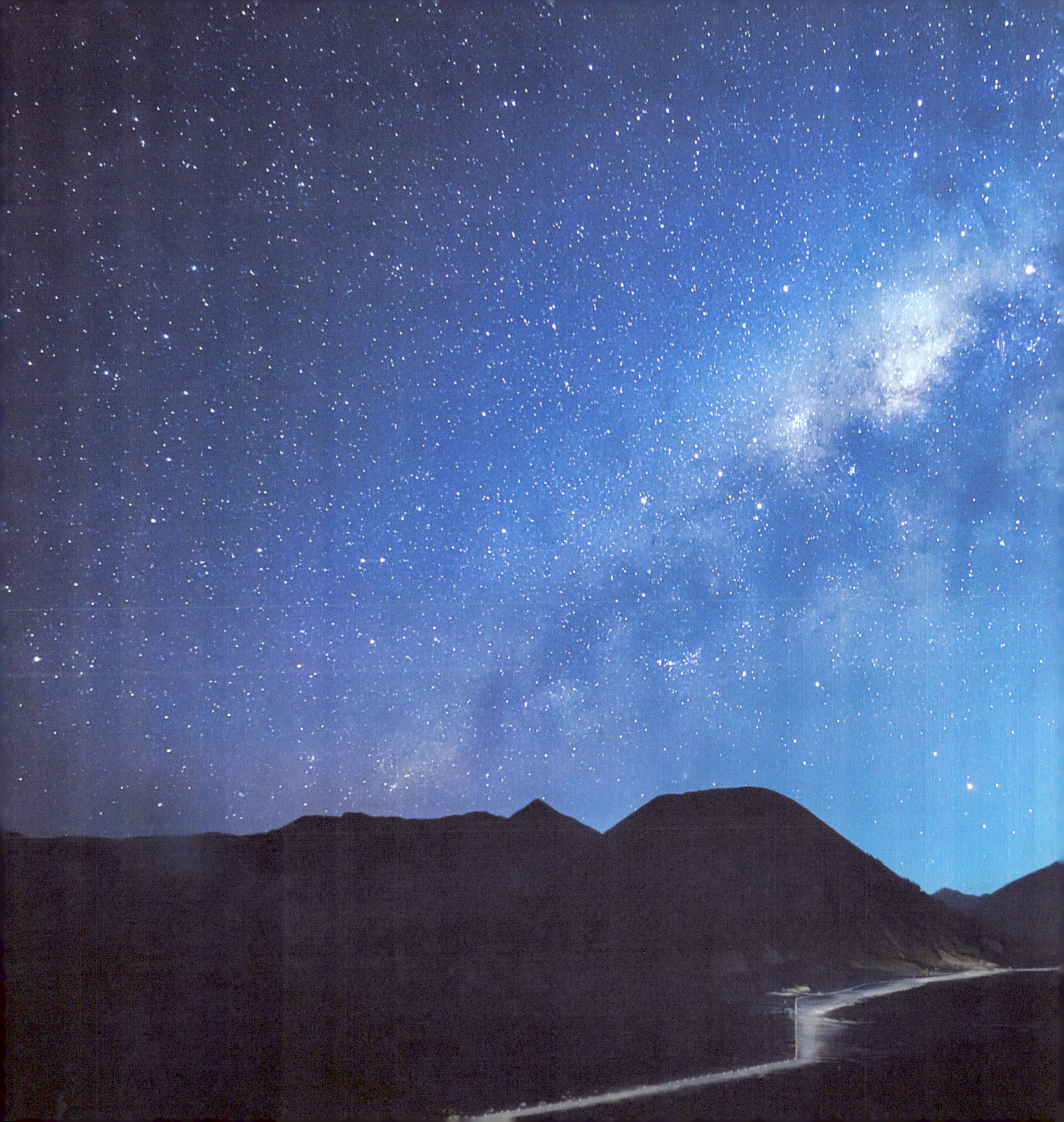

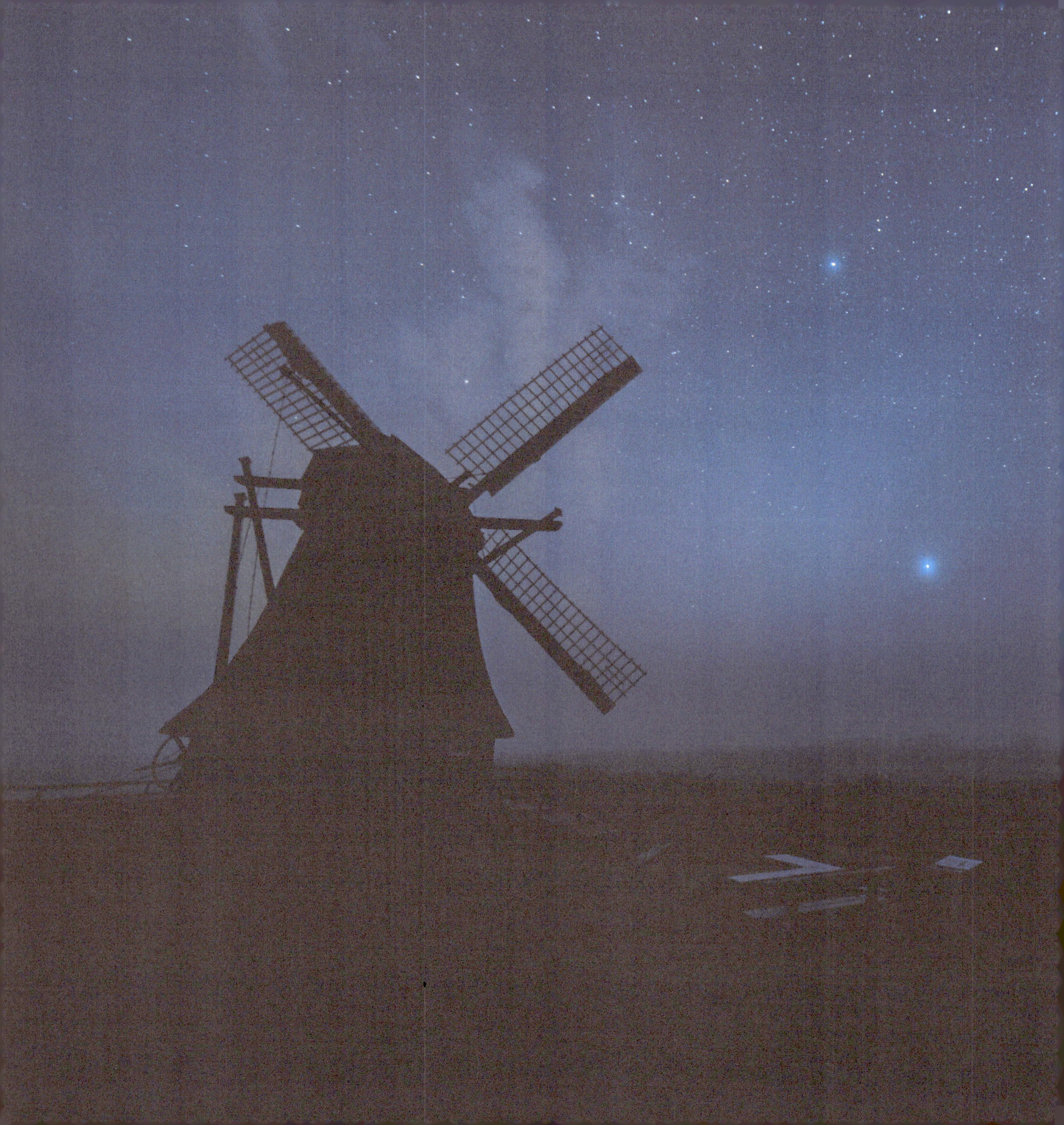

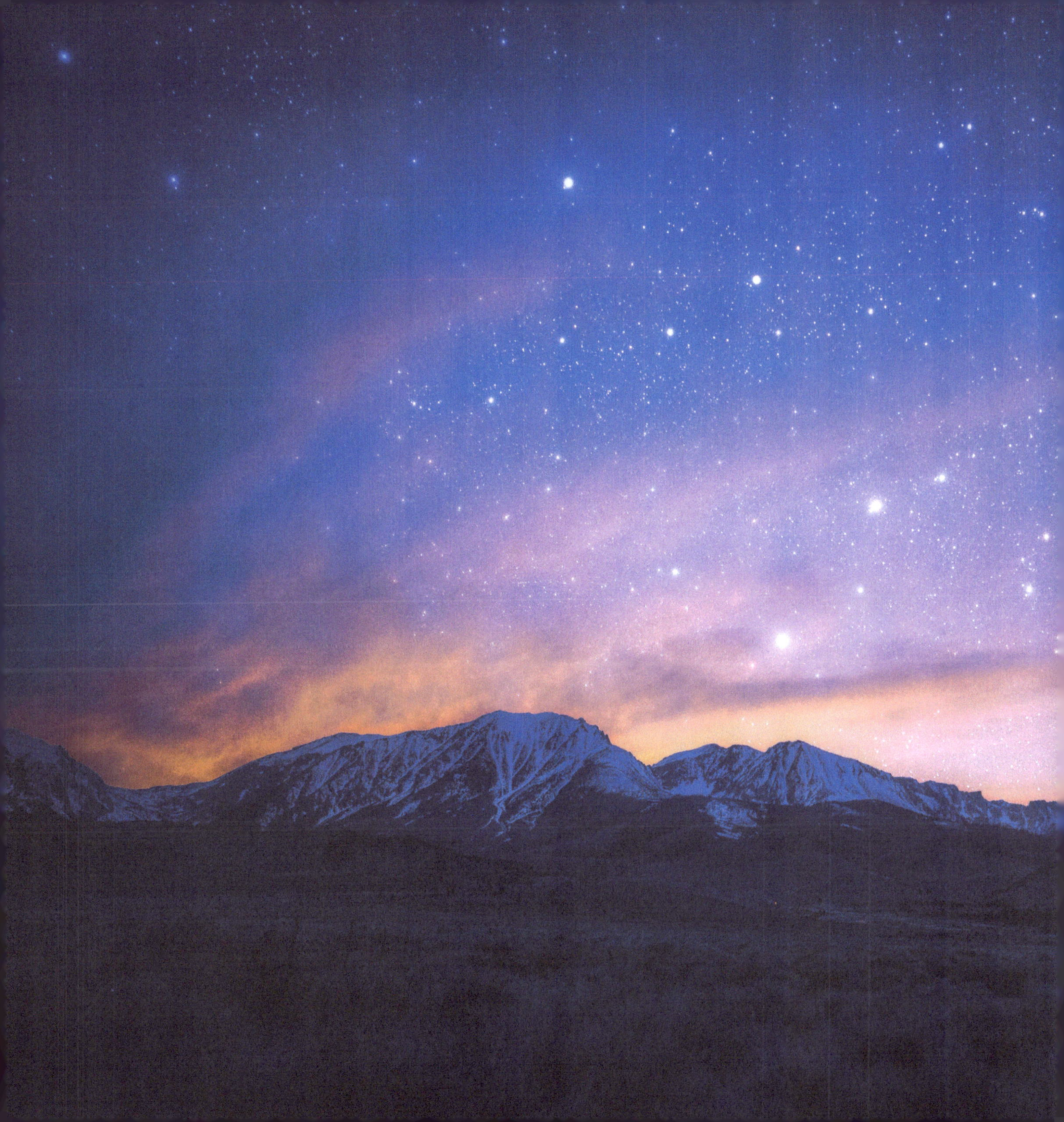

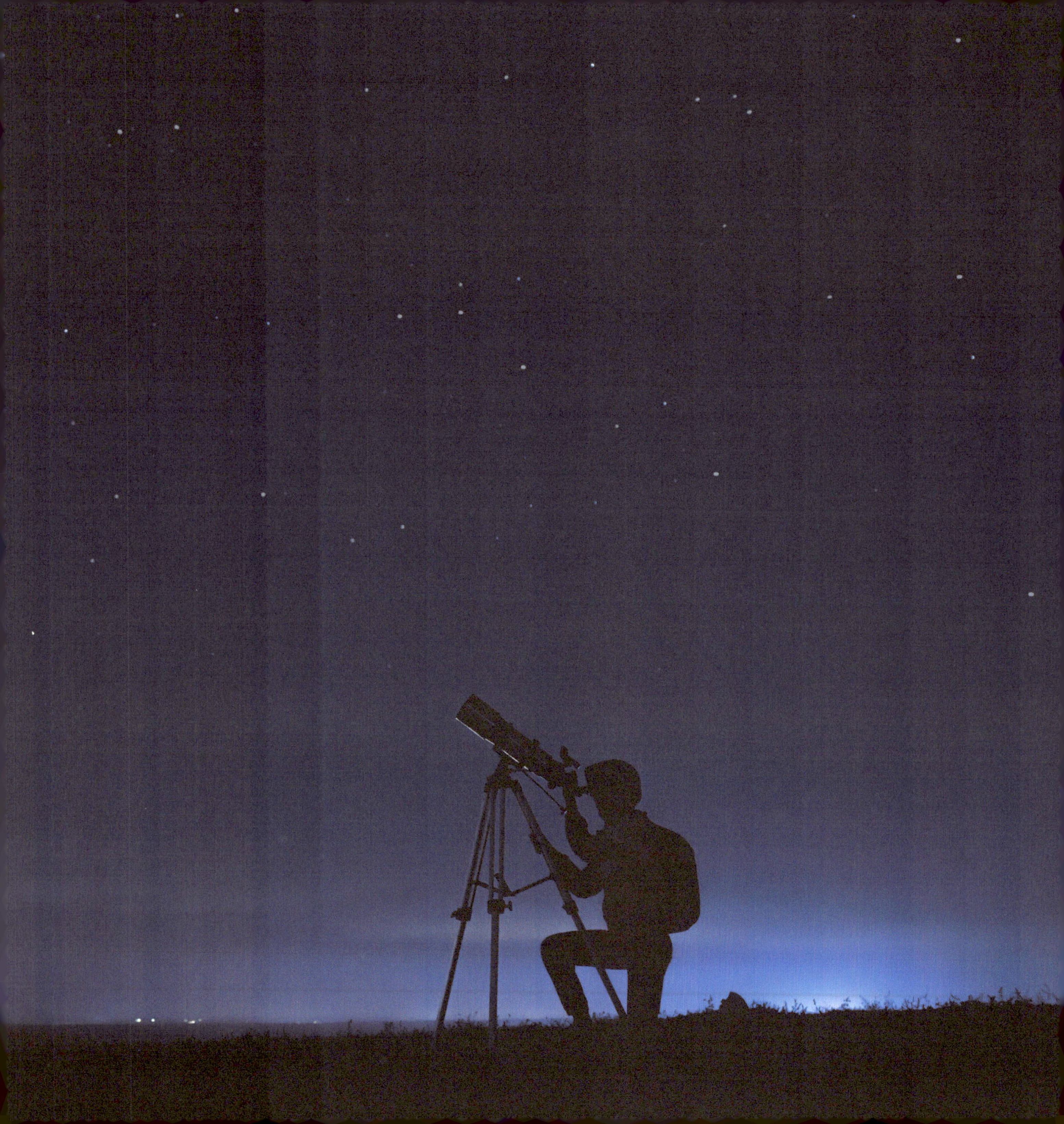

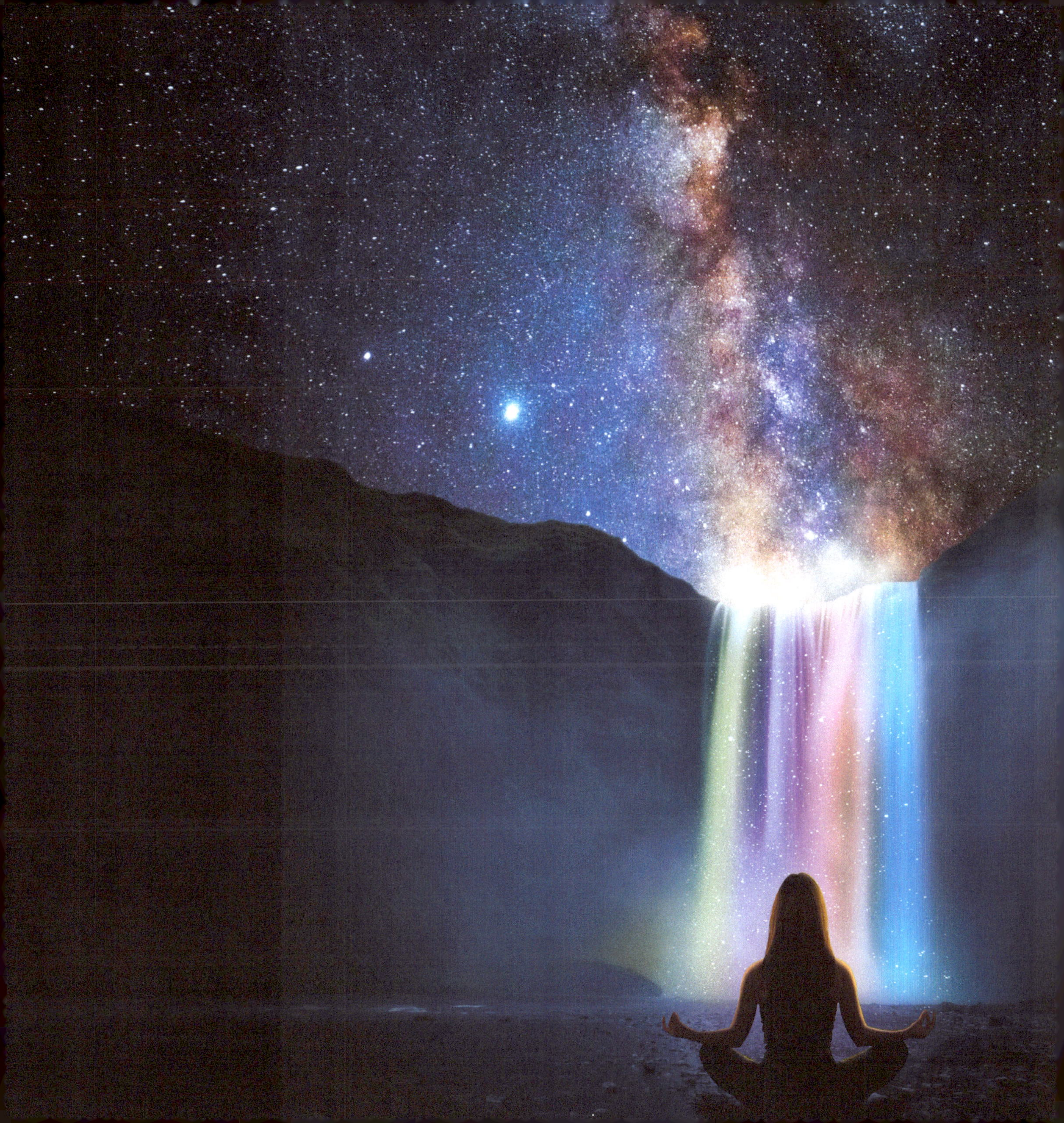

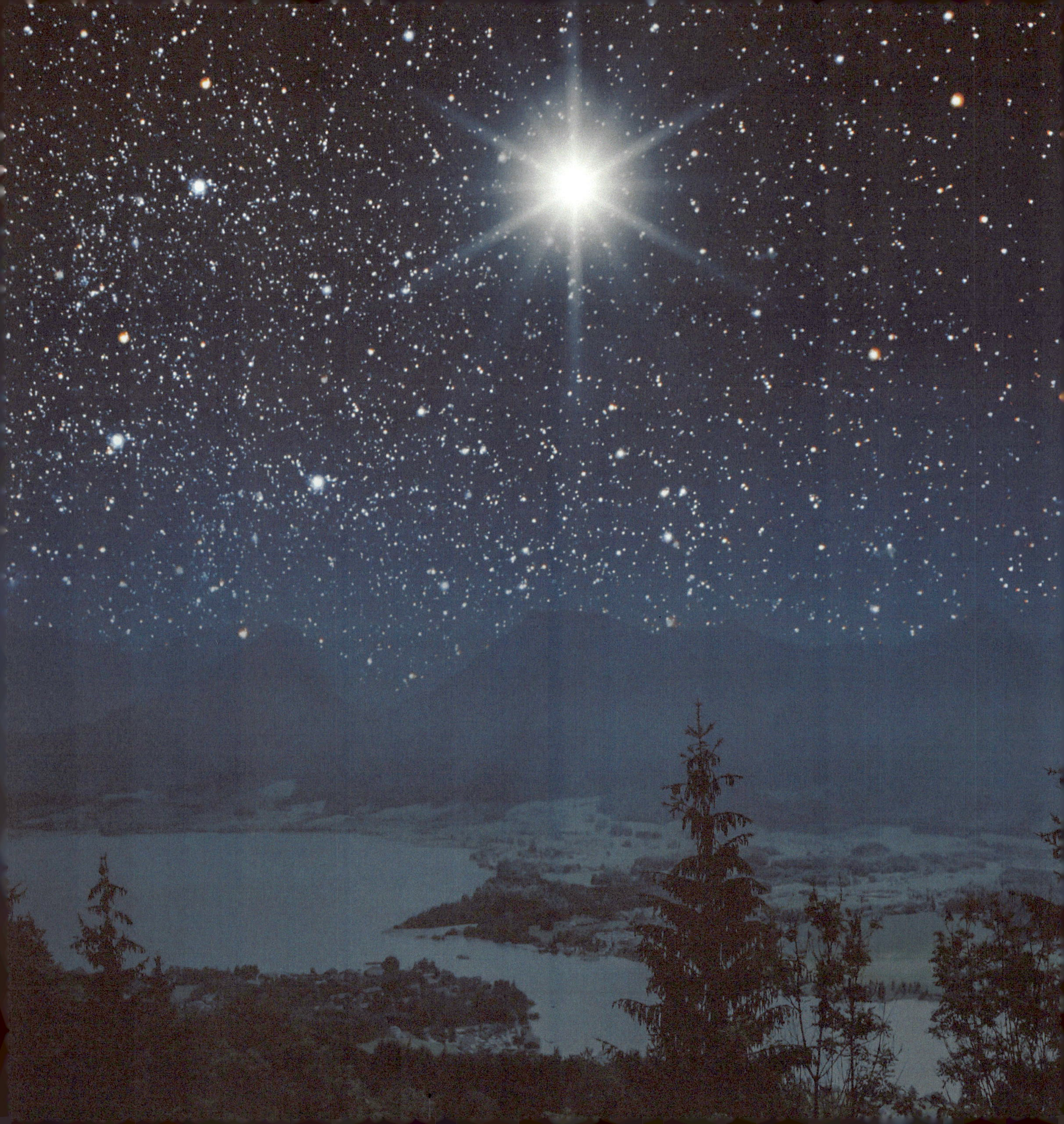

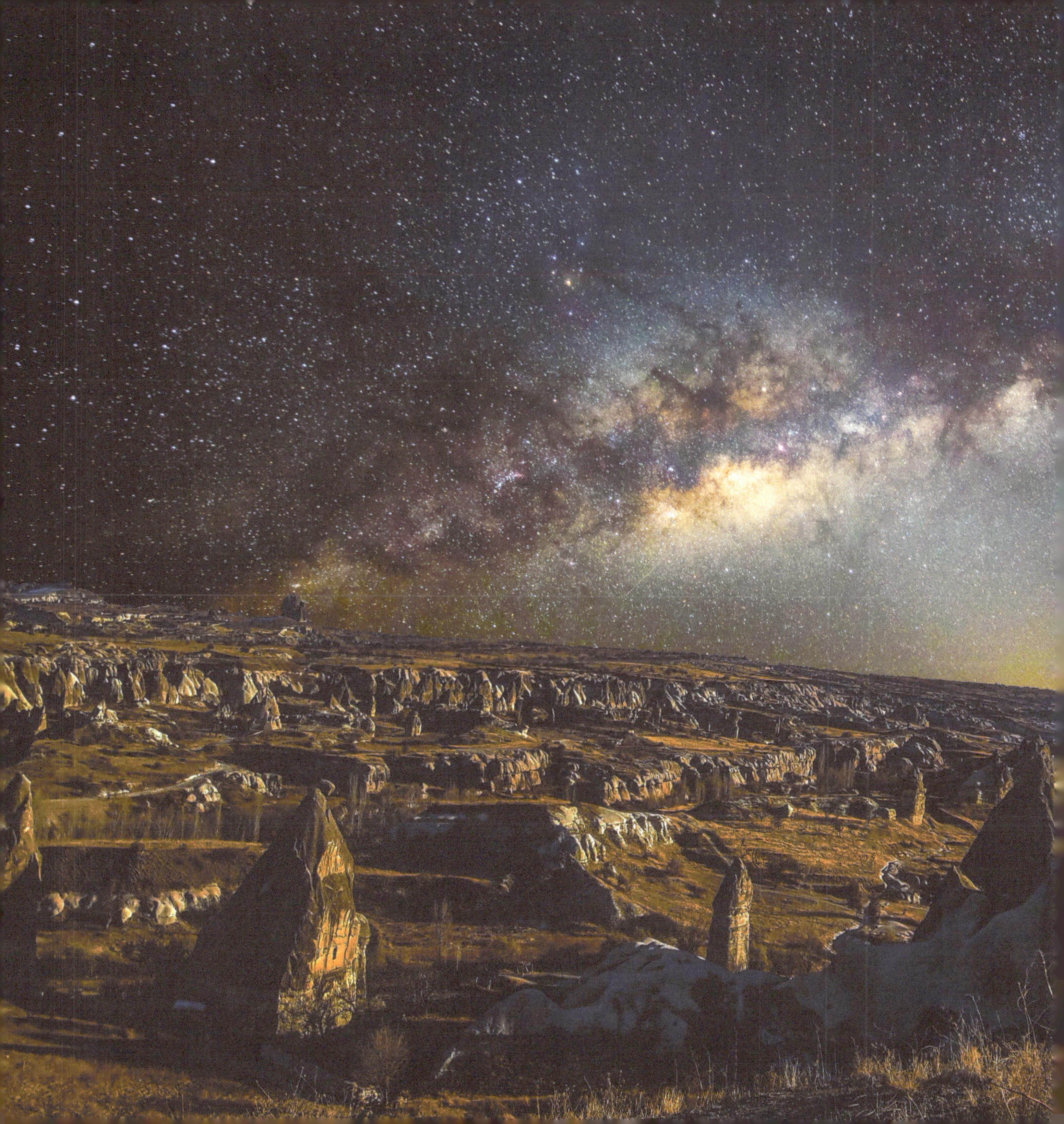

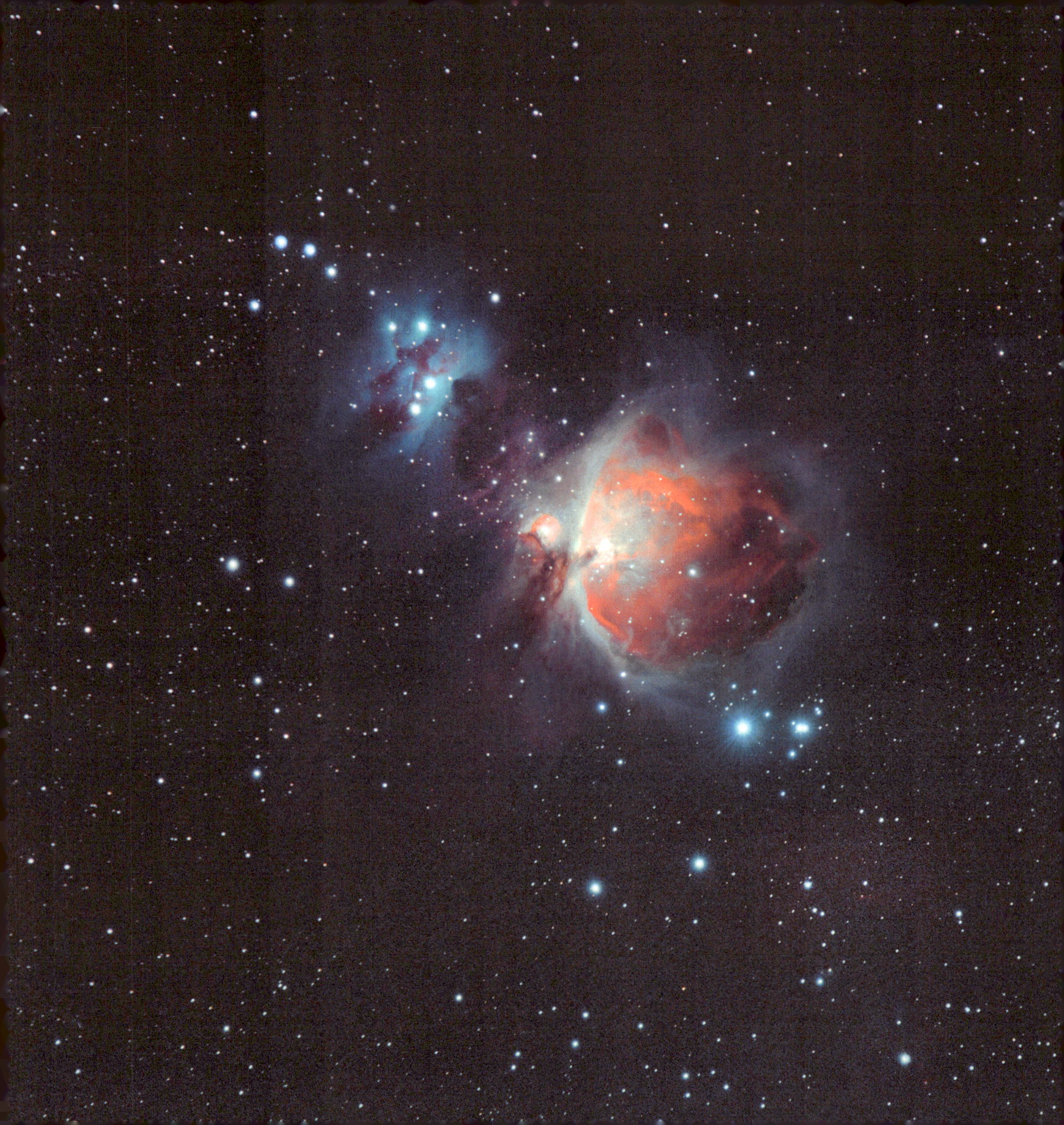

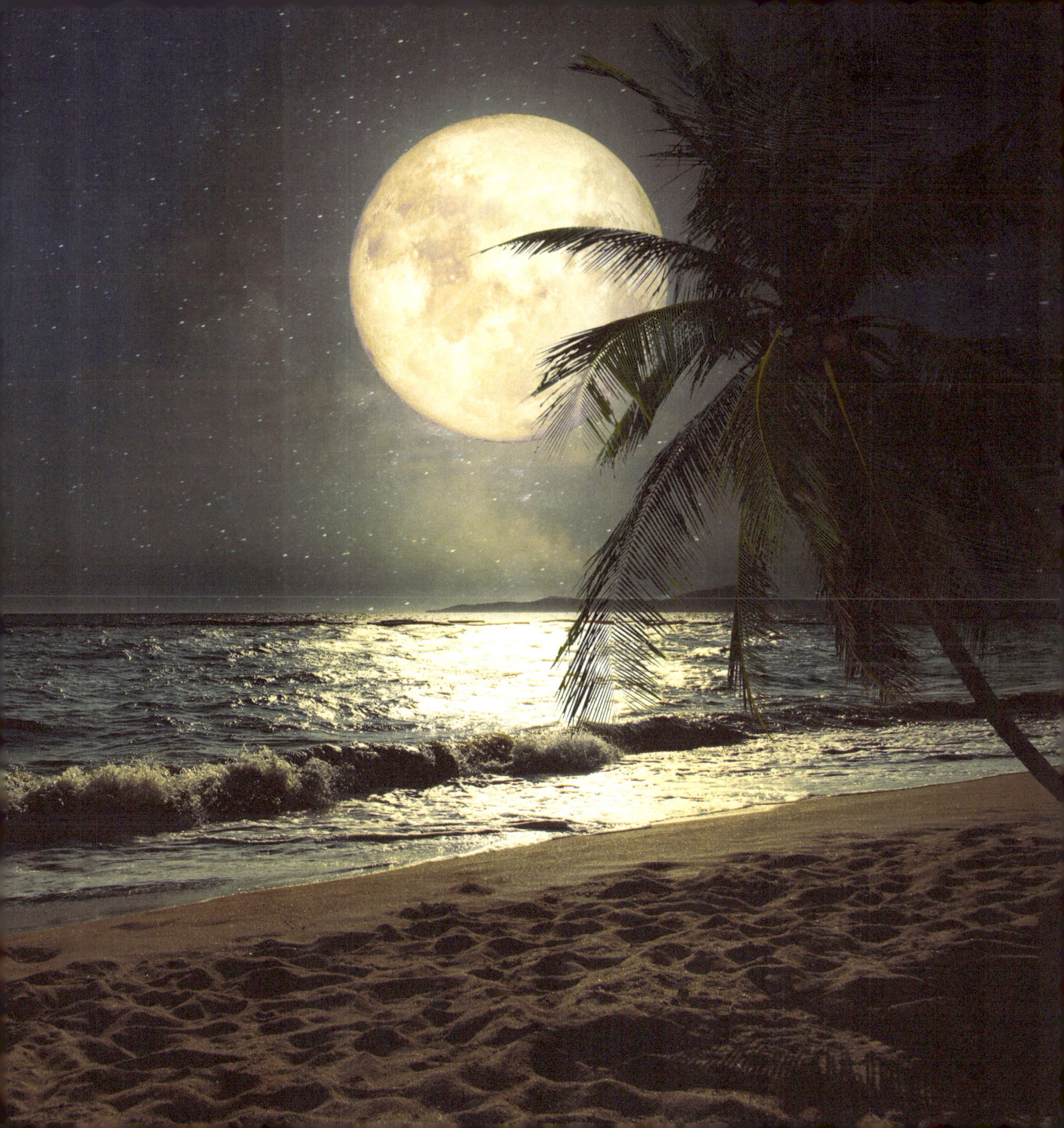

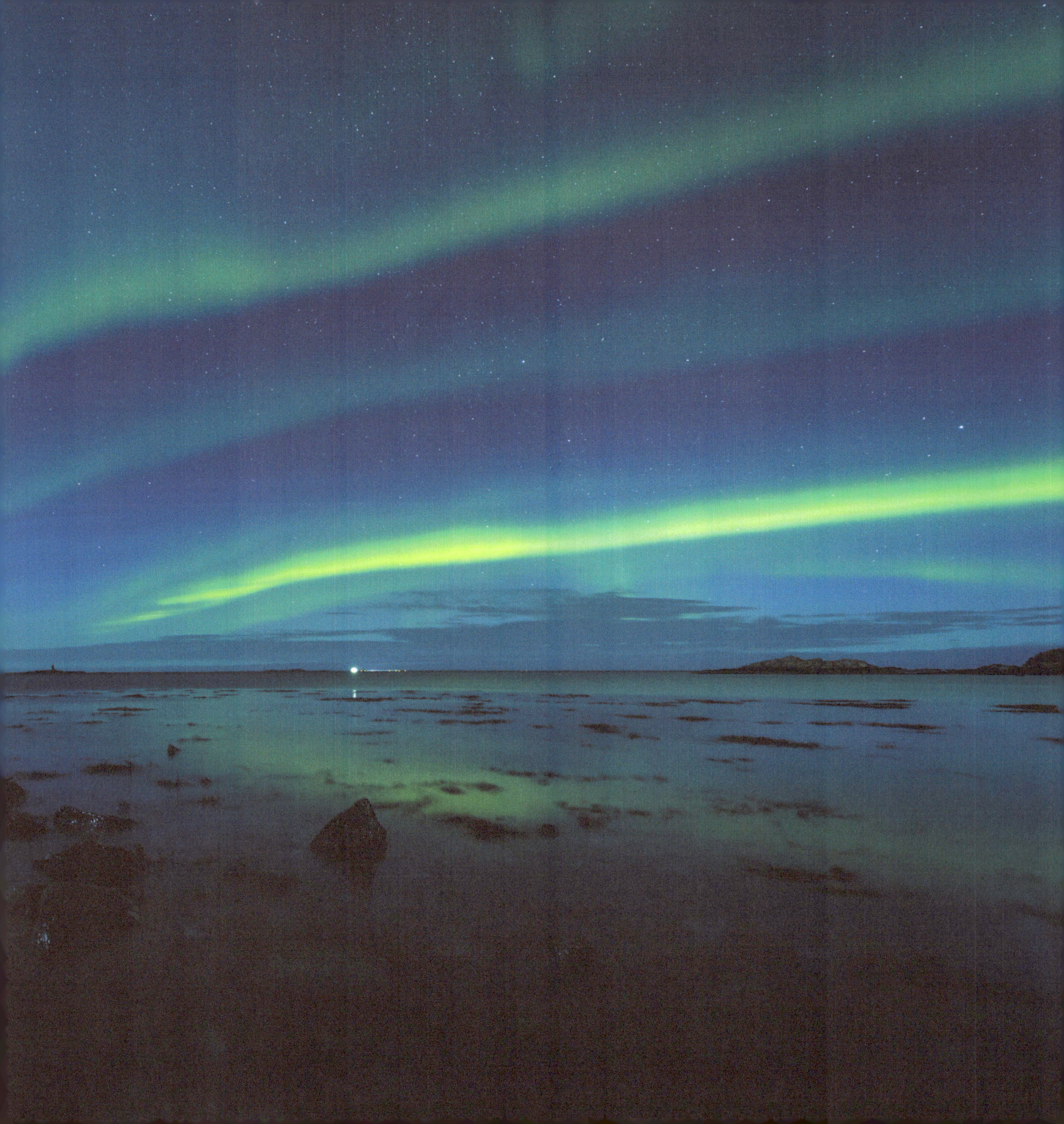

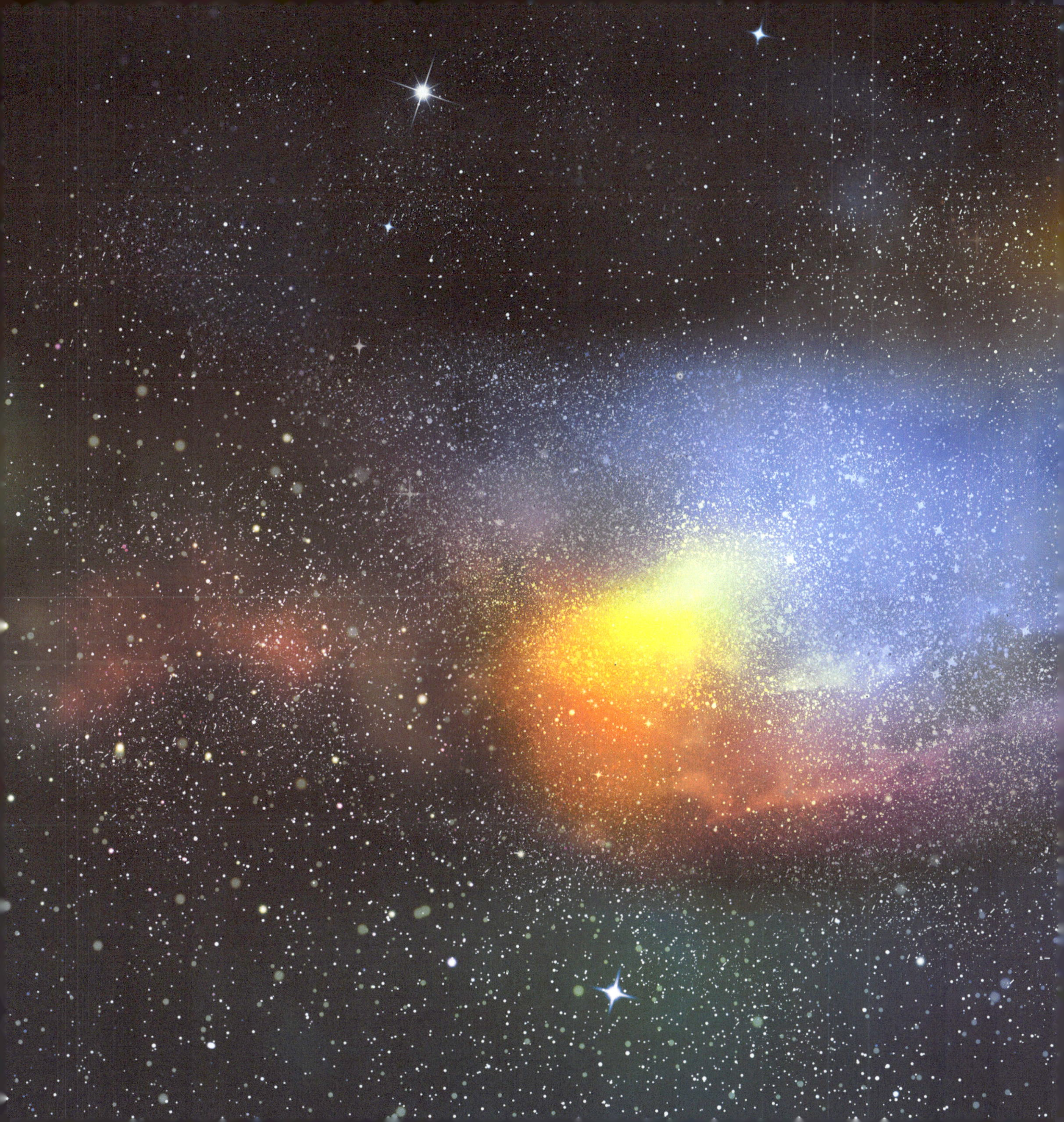

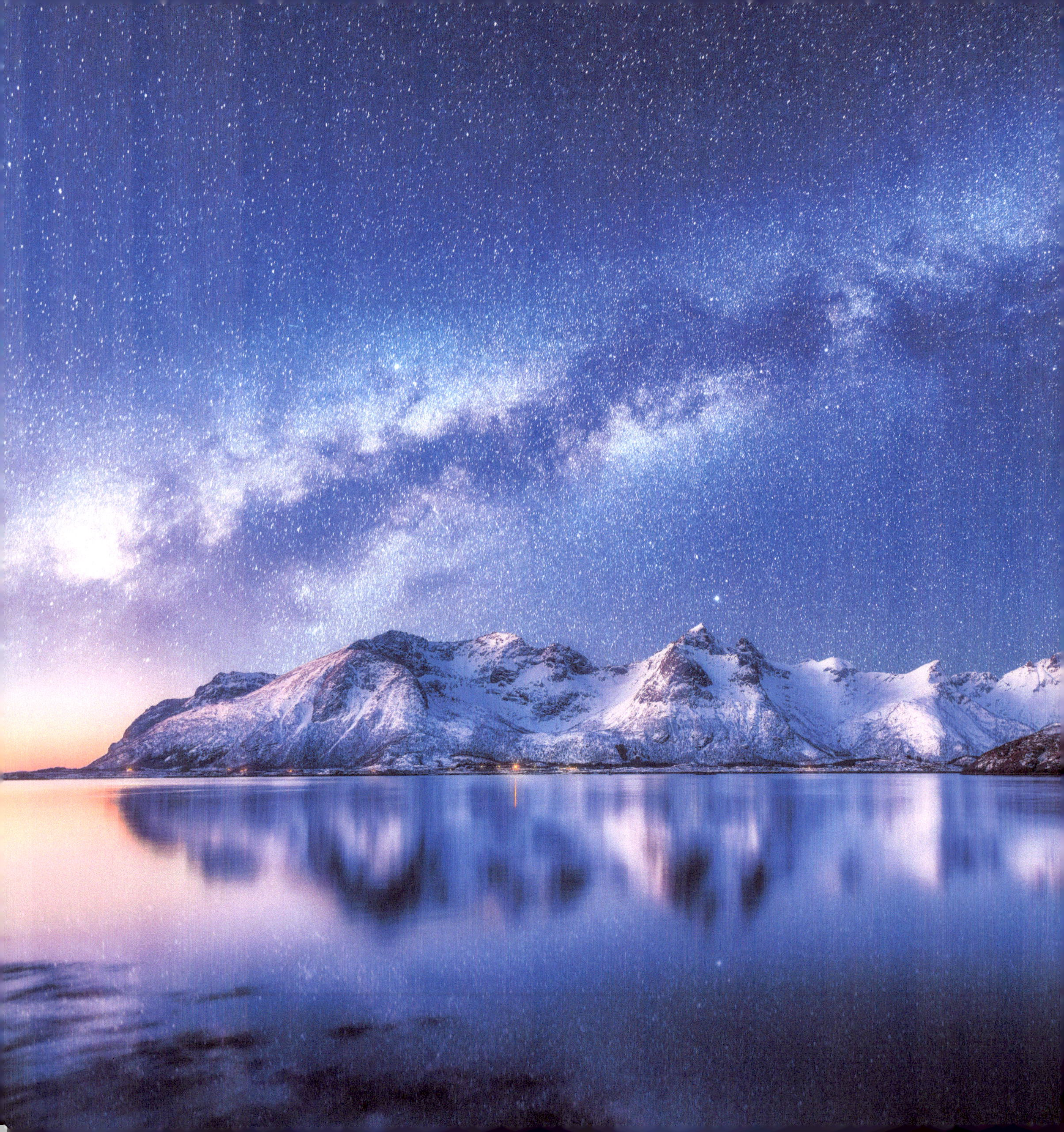

Lightning Source UK Ltd.
Milton Keynes UK
UKHW020631011222
413022UK00003B/199

* 9 7 9 8 7 4 4 9 3 8 9 0 1 *